Contents

Editorial

Why have development policy-makers, practitioners, and researchers been slow to recognise the contribution, needs – and rights – of older and younger people, in both South and North? The overemphasis of mainstream development on young and middle-aged adults is understandable to some extent, since it is at this stage of life that both women and men are physically and mentally mature, become parents, and are most capable of work. However, as articles here show, this is only part of the picture. An enormous contribution, including both paid and unpaid work, is made to all our societies by the young and the old. If these groups were better represented in civil service, government, and development funding agencies (all institutions that replicate the age and gender biases of surrounding society), policy might reflect reality more accurately.

Older women and young girls, in particular, make a contribution to household, community, and national development that is not only undervalued by their own households and communities, but ignored by policy-makers who assume them to be dependants, cared for by their families. 'One of the most overpowering myths in contemporary development thinking and strategies is that women and children do not work' (Sohoni 1995, 117).

Sustainable human development depends not only on recognising and supporting women in their social and economic roles, but on recognition of, and support for, the contribution of younger and older people of both sexes.

Articles here focus on a wide range of topics relating to gender, age, and generation. These include women's life histories, reproductive health education of adolescents, trafficking of young girls, the survival strategies of child-headed and grandparent-headed households affected by HIV/AIDS, older women's marginalisation from community-based organisations (CBOs), and the attitudes of older women and men to living alone or entering care homes when they reach the point where support is needed. Articles examining the issues facing older women and men slightly outnumber those that focus on the younger generation. Articles on other key aspects – such as girls' formal education, and harmful traditional practices, including child marriage – can be found in recent issues of *Gender and Development*, on Education and Training, and Violence Against Women.[1] It is hoped to include articles on child soldiers in a future issue on Humanitarian Work, to be published in 2001.

The girl child

Within the family, age and sex decide clout and both work against the girl child. Consequently, the girl is twice denied because of her age and gender, and she is twice removed from the benefits and entitlements of her childhood as well as her labour (Sohoni 1995, 124).

There is, now, widespread awareness among development workers and researchers that promoting girls' health and education is critical to development: it has economic and health benefits for the individual, but also for her family and community. A typical argument runs: 'If girls are not viewed by families and societies as having critical roles and potential for adulthood, and if opportunities are not available, then they will become mothers with children who are more likely to die in infancy, less healthy, less educated and less confident, and the cycle will be repeated. An investment in girls should be considered an investment in national development' (Kurz and Prather 1995, 5).

Girls are often less healthy than their brothers in poor households, where more resources are allocated to boys. Girls are less likely to be taken to clinics when they are unwell, and less likely to receive a good diet. In extreme situations, where the contribution of girl children is undervalued and their cost to the household seems unbearably high, they may suffer deliberate neglect in childhood, or be killed or allowed to die in infancy (Sohoni 1995). The phenomena of son preference and daughter neglect, combined with the toll that gender-based discrimination takes on women throughout their lives, have resulted in 100 million 'missing' women world-wide (Summers 1994, quoted in Leach 1998, 9).

There are 42 million fewer girls than boys enrolled in primary schools across the world. South Asia and sub-Saharan Africa have the widest gender gaps. In both regions, improvement is coming far too slowly. The proportion of girls in South Asian primary schools increased by only 2 per cent in the first half of the 1990s. Even when girls are enrolled, they are less likely than boys to complete their schooling.

However, there is relatively little awareness of the complex reasons that prevent millions of young girls worldwide from receiving education. It is more than poverty at household level, or even lack of provision, that prevents these girls from being educated. Attention to the ways in which gender and age come together to create disadvantage shows us that barriers to girls' education are concerned with the role that young girls are expected to play at present, and in the future.

Within the household, young girls are expected to substitute for their mothers if the latter are unable to perform the household duties that go with being female. This happens either during the day, preventing girls from attending school, or after school hours, preventing them from undertaking private study or making them too exhausted to continue their double role. Feminist critiques of existing development models, which focus on integrating women into production, have long pointed out the cost to girls of policies that only promote women's production, without challenging the gender division of labour within the home: 'If women are encouraged, or obliged by economic crisis, to spend ever-increasing hours in production, someone has to be found to compensate for the loss of labour within the home. This has had a serious negative impact on girl children' (Sen and Grown 1987, 43).

Currently, there is increasing pressure on children to labour outside the home, as well as inside – and this leads many children to be exploited (Chambers, preface to Johnson et al 1998). Parents need to boost family earnings, and employers know they can depress production costs by employing children and paying them lower wages.

In 1997, UNICEF estimated that there were at least 190 million child income-earners in the world (Johnson et al. 1998, 126). It is widely recognised that poverty means that many children need to work to survive, but coercive and exploitative forms of work – sex work, armed combat, or manual labour which stunts children's growth – must be replaced by employment that is non-exploitative, combined with an opportunity for education and training. In the United Nations Convention on the Rights of the Child (1989), widely ratified by countries across the world, children are declared to have the 'right to a childhood' – a specific period of the life course where learning, through schooling and play, should be uppermost.

There has been much energy expended by governments and NGOs throughout the world on curtailing child labour, but it seems clear that for many children and families there is no alternative. Poverty indicators are worsening in many countries in South and North, and many families are coping with the impact of economic crisis on employment and income generation by sending young and middle-aged adults to work away from impoverished regions. In communities in Africa, Asia, and Latin America, parents and breadwinners may be absent for another reason: as a result of AIDS. In her article, Judith Appleton discusses the coping strategies of households headed by children – and grandparents – in fishing communities in Tanzania. These children are replacing the productive capacity of their parents, by becoming fishers and farmers themselves. The opportunity for education is light years away from these boys and girls.

Adolescents, sexuality, and abuse

The second group of barriers to girls' education is related to the assumption that their only future role is as wives and mothers. If there is a long distance to travel to school, if classes are mixed-sex, if teachers are male, if learning materials challenge gender norms – all of these things may expose girls to possible sexual activity, abuse, and pregnancy. This will devalue them as future brides, and they may face a future of poverty and insecurity as a result. In contexts where employment opportunities are few, it is hard – even for loving and responsible parents – to risk these things in the hope that a girl may be able to make her own living through paid work at the end of her education.

In her article, Sabina Faiz Rashid of the major Bangladeshi NGO, BRAC, focuses on the Adolescent Reproductive Health Education (ARHE) programme, which teaches reproductive health and gender awareness in BRAC's own schools. These have been set up for adolescents who have not had the opportunity to attend school previously. BRAC seeks to reach girls and boys before they experiment sexually and place themselves at risk of pregnancy and sexually transmitted disease. The ARHE inculcates the idea that there is an alternative to early marriage and childbearing, for both girls and boys. It hopes to promote more equitable relations between the sexes, influencing families and communities.

Adolescent girls are widely stereotyped as potential sexual partners, pure and simple: their capacity to take on many different roles and tasks in society is ignored. As sexual partners, they may be acquired through fair means or foul. Culturally sanctioned forms of violence may be used against them, including forced or early marriage, genital mutilation, and forms of sexual slavery. In their article, Pratima Poudel and Jenny Carryer trace the origins of trafficking of girls in Nepal to a history of providing young girls to the monarch. They move on to present a critique of the current response of the Nepalese government and development-funding agencies to the shocking plight of trafficked Nepalese girls. After appalling abuse in the brothels of India and other 'receiving' countries, increasing numbers of young girls are being returned to Nepal to die of AIDS. Ostracised by their communities in poverty-stricken rural areas, many continue selling sex as their sole means of livelihood.

Young women's experience of employment

If young girls are married in adolescence, they become wives and mothers before they can experience independent adulthood. However, some do manage to break away from gender norms to take up income-generating activities or paid employment. Two articles in this collection examine different experiences of this nature. Rachel Slater's article is based on research into the life stories of four South African women who migrated to Cape Town during different eras and with different kinds of family ties and obligations. Two of the women she talked to arrived at a young age and survived on their wits, 'seeking social and financial independence from their families in the city' (Slater, this issue).

Rachel Slater points out that young unmarried women with no children are able to adapt to changing economic and social circumstances much better than those who have responsibility for children. As a result, many employers are now recruiting young women to work in factories and offices, in contexts as different as the export industries of Mexico and the telephone call centres of Europe. While much attention has been given to exploitative wages and conditions that this type of employment may involve, in the eyes of the young women workers themselves many jobs are liberating. In her article, Mary Kawar of the International Labour Organization (ILO) turns the focus away from what young women can offer the world of work, to what the world of work can offer young women. She analyses the impact of paid work on young women in Amman, Jordan,

and argues that it can enable them to challenge gender relations (although in a limited way) within their families. They are living proof that education and employment really can create a new 'life-stage' for women.

Recognising the labour of older women

The world of older people – in particular, the world of the 'old old', aged 80 and over – is a predominantly female world. Throughout the world, male life-expectancy is lower than that for women. While social issues may be a factor in some contexts, there is also a universal biological cause. Older populations are thus predominantly composed of widowed females. In 1981, in India, the average time that a man could expect to be a widower was 6.2 years; for a woman, widowhood lasted an average 11.5 years (Owen 1996, 148).

The year 1999 was designated the United Nations International Year for the Older Person. The invisibility of older people from development debates is a grave mistake in economic and social terms: the contribution that these groups make to human welfare and development is huge, and could be even greater. In their article focusing on three low-income urban communities in Lima, Peru, Fiona C Clark and Nina Laurie state that elderly people – and in particular women – have contributed much to the rise of social movements in Peru. Their article, like two others in this collection, reflects the progress made in parts of Latin America and the Caribbean towards addressing the needs of older people. In this region, it has been argued, 'perhaps the role that so many Latin American and Caribbean women at midlife and older play within their families and within society can serve as our example and our guide. Steered by this, we can pursue solutions that are less "medicalised", more humanitarian, and more caring' (Guerra de Macedo, in PAHO/AARP 1989, viii).

However, this hope is not always achieved. In their article, Clark and Laurie argue that the feminist movement in Peru has been surprisingly slow to adopt the concerns of older women into its agenda. They argue that the very same organisations that have benefited from older women's activities – and leadership in the past – refuse to see them as legitimate beneficiaries of welfare in very old age.

In old age, as in earlier stages of life, gender stereotypes operate. Women who are past their childbearing years are seen as less useful and less attractive as marital partners. Commonly, widows are not allowed to marry again, but sometimes (as in parts of Southern Africa) they are 'inherited' by the male relatives of the deceased husband (Chitsike 1995). Inheritance laws that pass on possessions, including land, through the male line will by-pass widows, but customary practices obliging relatives to support them may have been eroded, while income-generating opportunities may be hard to come by. There are relatively high levels of illiteracy among older women, and the education offered to generations born in the first third of the twentieth century tended to reinforce, rather than challenge, ideas of them as wives and mothers (Owen 1996). In short, 'female poverty at the end of life is a consequence of all the inequalities a woman has endured since birth' (ibid, 163).

In her article, Sylvia Beales of HelpAge International draws on her organisation's research and work around the world, to highlight similarities in the experience of older women in poor communities. She asks: 'While longevity is in many ways a triumph of social development, if it means that women and men are growing older without becoming any less poor, and that they undergo additional years of struggle for daily survival, can we really claim that this is social progress?' (Beales, this issue).

While efforts are made by development policy-makers to integrate women and girls living in poverty into the labour market as a solution to poverty, this does not generally happen with older women. Older women are assumed either to be supported by their families, or – in all post-industrialised countries and in some 'developing' countries – to have a pension to fall back on. However, neither of these is a guarantee of security in later life. In situations of extreme poverty, families often do not have adequate income to support an extra member, and need a pension to help with survival: in some situations, an older person's pension may ensure survival for their entire family. However, access to pensions depends on one's gender identity. Fiona Clarke and Nina Laurie's article traces the ways in which pension reforms and cutbacks have affected women. They point out that the gendered division of labour makes it very hard for women to make all the personal contributions required of them. As a result, in Peru, 99.6 per cent of all those who lack their own pension and rely on that of a spouse are women (Clarke and Laurie, this issue).

Countering negative stereotypes of old age

Older people themselves – and women in particular – are influenced by the negative stereotypes about old age that surround them. In their article, Jacquie Cheetham and Wendy Alba examine a participatory research exercise carried out by two organisations working in the Dominican Republic. The article has several lessons for policy-makers. These include the fact that negative images of old age and older people abound, and that older people themselves are as likely to equate positive qualities with youth as young people are. Respect for older people is being eroded in the current era of rapid social and economic change, and 'globalisation' of culture as well as the economy.

One of the most interesting findings is that the older people in the Santo Domingo study emphasised their need for education.

Most policy-makers tend to focus either on the education of children, or non-formal education or training for adults. It is clear from this article that older people have a very clear idea of what education can do for them, in terms of enabling them to contribute more to society, ensure their own economic stability, and organise in political groupings. The older people involved in this research have since become an active political force for change, organising classes, political activities, and welfare support, from the first community centre for older women in Santo Domingo.

Older women in the research saw their interests in terms of family wellbeing, and tended not to see themselves as individuals with separate needs. Many equated their needs with those of their families. In their article on urban Mexico, Maribel Blasco and Ann Varley focus on the relatively high number of older women – one in ten of the over-sixties – who are living alone rather than with their families or in institutions. Older people in developing countries are much more likely to live with their families; for example, in Brazil and Hong Kong, around half the elderly live in extended families (United Nations 1995, 4). However, Blasco and Varley encountered some older women who seemed to prefer solitude and insecurity to continuing to care for households and grandchildren into their later years.

Like older women, older men face difficulties rooted in social expectations of them connected with their gender identity. Many suffer from their inability to live up to the widespread stereotypes of them as family breadwinners. Maribel Blasco and Ann Varley found that people pitied older men who were on their own, since they had lost their identity as breadwinners. (Of course, it should be said that not all younger men live up to this social expectation of them!) Older men who are unable to contribute are marginalised and abused. Sylvia Beales also discusses this in her article, arguing that work to address older men's issues needs to be considered a part of 'gender and development' work.

Life histories and generation

Rachel Slater's article looks at the collecting of life histories as a method of development research and a way of assessing the impact of particular trends or events on various people, thereby informing future development policy. Since society changes around us, our choices are different from those of our mothers or daughters. In Cape Town, the context of her research, the political upheavals and legal changes of the apartheid regime meant that luck played a part in determining different women's chances of survival and stability. As individuals, we are shaped not only by our age, gender, and other aspects of social identity, but also by the unique times and events through which we live, at a particular stage of our life course.

Conclusion

We all acquire valuable experience and understanding in the course of our lives, and this should shape development analysis and policy.

All writers here argue that younger and older people cannot be assumed to be dependent on the generation in-between. Gender analysis allows researchers and policy-makers to investigate who does what in households and communities, how time is used, and what different people gain from their work. Similar methods can be used to determine the contribution of different generations, and these must be sensitive to gender issues too. The fact that young children and very old people have welfare needs must not be forgotten, but equally it is critical to recognise the young and the elderly – and in particular girls and older women – as economic contributors. Just as women's work is made invisible by conventional assumptions about male breadwinners, the labour of children and older people is obscured by social norms which treat them as dependants.

As stated above, different people gain different things from their work. Gender and development approaches demonstrate that there is a link between the recognition of one's contribution and the degree to which one is then able to eat, rest, and – crucially – participate in decision-making at many different levels. Older people are more commonly acknowledged than children to have the 'right' to participate in decision-making, but even this is not often respected in development policy and practice. Sylvia Beales' article lists many different suggestions for ways in which her organisation is considering ensuring the active participation of older people in development policy-making, to everyone's benefit. Increasing interest in the principle of involving children in development policy-formulation can also be seen: 'We risk more than adversely affecting the quality of children's lives by not listening to their voices and views. We risk missing out on the richness and innovative perspectives that can be offered by children and young people of varying experiences and from varying situations' (Johnson et al 1998, 4).

In conclusion, it is critically important that commitments to promoting the rights of children and older people to equality and development, made during the past 15 years, strengthen and are strengthened by a commitment to equality between males and females. It is gender stereotypes that send little boys into battle and banish older men into the bush when they can no longer be seen as breadwinners. It is gender stereotypes that lead older women to labour inside the home, doing work that is invisible to the outside world and undervalued by their own families. In addition to having this contribution recognised and valued through policies designed to address over-work and exploitation, policy is needed that will eradicate the extreme poverty experienced by many young and old people, and end prejudice against them.

Notes

1 *Gender and Development*, Vol. 6, No. 2, 1998, and *Gender and Development*, Vol. 6,: No. 3, 1998.

References

Chitsike C (1995) 'NGOs, gender, culture and multiculturalism: a Zimbabwean perspective', in *Gender and Development* Vol 3, No.1

Johnson, V, Ivan-Scott, E, Gordon, G, Pridmore, P, and Scott, P (eds) (1998) *Stepping Forward: Children and young people in the development process*, IT Publications, UK

Kurz K and Prather C (1995) *Improving the Quality of Life of Girls*, UNICEF, USA

Leach F (1998) 'Gender, education and training: an international perspective' in *Gender and Development*, Vol. 6, No. 2, Oxfam GB, UK

Owen M (1996) *A World of Widows*, Zed Books, UK

PAHO (Pan-American Health Organisation)/AARP (American Association of Retired Persons) (1989) *Mid-Life and Older Women in Latin America and the Caribbean*, PAHO/AARP/WHO, USA

Sen, G and Grown, C (1987) *Development, Crises, and Alternative Visions: Third World Women's Perspectives*, Zed Books, UK

Sohoni, NK (1995) *The Burden of Girlhood: A global inquiry into the status of girls*, Third Party Publishing Company, USA

United Nations (1995) *The World's Women: Trends and statistics*, UN, USA

Why we should invest in older women and men:

the experience of HelpAge International

Sylvia Beales

In this article, I explore the roles of older women and men in the developing world, and the barriers they encounter in the course of contributing to their families and communities. Older women face multiple disadvantages arising from gender-based prejudice, the heavy burden of manual and reproductive labour that they bear, and the longevity of females in comparison to males. Discrimination against women needs world-wide acknowledgement and action; yet, as is argued here, it is important to broaden our analysis of gender issues. Many men, too, face marginalisation, as the ageing process undermines their ability to provide for their families.

Currently, the world is undergoing profound demographic changes, which pose great challenges to development and social policy-makers. One of these changes is the growth in the number of older people in our societies. Old age has been typically seen as a phenomenon of developed countries, but, in fact, the great majority (two-thirds) of those over 60 years of age live in the developing world. This proportion is increasing steadily, due to improvements in health, hygiene, and basic services, and will reach nearly three-quarters by the 2030s (UNFPA and CBGS 1999). The US Bureau of the Census (Washington DC) calculates that by 2020 countries such as Cuba, Argentina, Thailand, and Sri Lanka will have higher proportions of older people than the US does today. By 2025, numbers of older people in the developing world are on course to double to 850 million, comprising 12 per cent of the global population.

The proportion of younger and older people is changing dramatically. Globally, the young still outnumbered the old by 7:1 in 1995, but this ratio is declining (UNFPA 1998, 13). In spite of the global challenge of HIV/AIDS, UN projections indicate that deaths from AIDS will change the young–old ratio in sub-Saharan Africa from 15:1 in 2000 to 4:1 in 2050 (UN 1996).

For many, old age is a period of chronic poverty and powerlessness. Throughout the world, older people are often economically poorer and suffer worse social and political exclusion than do other age groups. In developing countries, the problem is made worse, given that large numbers of people of all ages endure extreme poverty, which affects all aspects of their material and social existence. The cumulative effect of marginalisation and poverty throughout the life span is absolute poverty in old age.

While increased longevity is in many ways a triumph of social development, if it means that women and men are growing older without becoming any less poor, and that they undergo additional years of struggle for daily survival, can we really claim that this is social progress?

HelpAge International

The information in this article comes from research and programme experience in many developing countries, accumulated by HelpAge International (HAI). HAI is a world-wide network of local and national organisations in the developing and developed world, which works with disadvantaged older people on issues of poverty, rights, and exclusion. HAI aims to make a lasting improvement to the lives of older people, through supporting their empowerment, promoting their equality, and seeking to end discrimination against them. HAI is committed to the 18 United Nations Principles of Older Persons stated in UN Resolution 46/91, with their headings of Independence, Care, Self-Fulfilment, Dignity, and Participation.

Attention to the gender-based discrimination facing older women – and men – is an essential feature of HAI's programme and working practices. This means examining how cultural norms determine women's and men's social and economic power, and analysing how that power is inexorably reduced as people grow older. Deep-rooted negative attitudes towards older people are both the cause and the symptom of the problems routinely described by those we work with. Negative attitudes towards older people result in ageism, defined by HAI as a 'collective failure of individuals and organisations to provide a professional service to people because of their age'. The HAI definition continues: '[Ageism] can be detected in processes, attitudes, and behaviour which amount to discrimination through unwitting prejudice, ignorance, thoughtlessness and stereotyping which disadvantage older people' (HAI training course 1999). An example of this is the characterisation of older people as dependants. In fact, HelpAge International's participatory research in countries as different as St Lucia, Ghana, and South Africa has revealed that the majority of older people are net contributors to their families, rather than net recipients of support. It is only by understanding and valuing the contributions of women and men throughout their life-course that such attitudes and their related behaviours can be altered.

Issues faced by older women

Everyone cares for older relatives, but women do most of the work (Graham 2000)

The fact of women's greater longevity means that the world of older people is predominantly one of poor women, often widowed, who all too often face physical suffering, economic disadvantage, and social exclusion (Heslop 1999, De Haan 1998). Women currently outlive men in nearly all countries. The US Bureau of the Census forecasts that by 2025 the number of women aged over 60 in the developing world will increase by 150 per cent.

There are various theories to explain the growing difference between women and men's longevity, which is approximately 5–8 years in women's favour in the developed world, and 3–5 years in the developing world. Poverty studies in the West and parts of Eastern Europe argue that there are genetic differences, as well as socio-economic factors, that affect men's longevity more than women's, including men's greater exposure to industrial hazards, conflict-related deaths, and lifestyle choices such as alcoholism. Research (which comes in the main from the West) has established that older men are more likely to suffer from heart disease or a stroke than women, and are more likely to die from chronic respiratory disease than women (WHO 1999).

Older people themselves acknowledge that it is older women who are the most vulnerable, especially if they are widowed, childless, and in declining health. As an older woman from Bangladesh put it during HAI research, *'We are poor, we are old, we are women – so no one wants us. We are alone'* (HelpAge et al. 2000).

In HAI's experience, the concerns voiced by older women are similar to those of younger women. These are to maintain the good health of themselves and their family, and to provide for their own and their family's economic security, and their own care needs. Good health is critical for survival, and illness is expensive. However, a lifetime spent battling against the effects of poor nutrition, violence, onerous working conditions, multiple pregnancies, and lack of education means that many women are already in declining health when they reach old age. The burden of caring for the old still falls on female family members, often on women who are themselves ageing and in failing health.

Most older women continue to work into very old age: for personal survival, to support others, and for pleasure. Research in various contexts from Asia, Africa, and Latin America confirms that older women do not want to be dependent on their children or to cause them anxiety (Sim and Ree 1997, in the context of Korea). Many spend more time working than the men in their communities. Participatory research in Zanzibar, Tanzania, recorded that the daily rest period of older men in the community was approximately seven hours. In comparison, older women were occupied during those hours with multiple tasks, such as cooking, cleaning, fetching firewood, child-care, and pounding grain. Despite this, older women received few material benefits and had less control and ownership over income-generating activities than the men (Forrester 1999).

In addition to producing food or earning income themselves, many older women perform reproductive work at home, thereby freeing other family members to work outside the home. HAI participatory research in Lao revealed that older women continue to carry the greater burden of reproductive labour into very old age (Graham 2000). In many contexts, older women have a special responsibility for family care, including caring for the 'old old', and the sick and disabled. HAI's experience is that older women can demonstrate remarkable flexibility in adapting this role to new economic and social conditions. For example, they may take on additional care burdens for grandchildren, caused by the absence or death of their children (for example, through changing migration practices, or AIDS-related death), or changes in family structures caused by conflict and natural disasters. In addition, older women often organise themselves into groups, and become involved in community activities.

Older women may be rewarded for their industry by their children: in Ghana, for example, they have reported that their contribution was recognised by their being made the guardians of valuable cloth and seeds (Ahenkora 1999). However, in other cases, women may find themselves cast out. Inheritance laws that exclude women have a pernicious effect on older women, who forfeit land-based assets on being widowed. A respondent in the HelpAge International research in Bangladesh put the issue very starkly: *'If the house burns, residue remains; if the husband dies, nothing remains'* (HAI/BAAIGM et al 2000).

Religion and culture can also conspire to isolate older women, as a woman's status in many societies is very dependent on having a husband, and divorce or widowhood can lead to a woman spending the rest of her lifetime in misery (Owen 1999). Older widows rarely have the opportunity to marry again, and so their lives may be consigned to loneliness and much greater dependence on their children. Since they can no longer produce children, they may have also lost a major 'function' in the eyes of society (Forrester 1999). It is socially acceptable in most cultures for men to marry younger women, and this may lead to older wives being abandoned. In Tanzania, women rarely take their cases to court, for fear of reprisal and ridicule (ibid).

In HAI's experience, most of the older people who live alone are women. For example, in our research in Laos the figure was 73 per cent. Such women can experience extreme destitution. One older woman in Laos told the research team: *'It is hard for me to come and meet with you for three days, because I have to go to the forest to find food to eat and sell. If I don't go, I won't have any food to eat'* (Graham 2000, 27).

In Tanzania, witchcraft was raised as a key issue for older widows living alone: 'The solitude of a widow brings additional problems – if she is not seen much about the village, an air of mystery may grow up around her, which contributes strongly to accusations of being a witch. ... they are alone, so have no support to ward off the accusations, they are weak and vulnerable, they are poor, so do not have resources to fight, they are often seen as being cleverer than older men, they often have physical signs of being a witch, for example red eyes,[1] wrinkles, bags under the eyes, twisted limbs, gnarled hands' (Forrester 1999, 53).

Issues facing older men

While many projects in HAI's international programme explicitly target older women, both as 'clients' and as agents of change, we have not to date been sufficiently thorough in applying a gender analysis to men's experience of ageing.

The economic roles assigned to males from early youth mean that the loss of earning power has serious consequences for men's position in society. In youth and middle age, many men are household heads, and are seen (accurately or not) as the main breadwinners for their families. Evidence from HAI participatory research and project experience in all regions

suggests that men's power is conferred by this productive capacity. The studies show that the status that accompanies men's productive role does not automatically transfer to the older man. A report from Bolivia, from organisations working with HAI, states that older men who are no longer producing a recognised income for the household are given 'the smallest plate of food and left outside the house in the cold for hours'. In Bangladesh, a story is told of a disabled grandfather who is being removed from the family home in a basket by the son, so that the 'burden' of the old man can be disposed of in the forest. On seeing this, the grandson observes, *'Father, please be sure to bring back the basket'.* On being asked why by the father, the grandson replies: *'Because I will need it when you grow old'* (HAI/BAAIGM et al 2000, 15).

This story justifies the anxiety of many older men as they become increasingly less able to earn income. Employers may be unwilling to hire an older man, who may be illiterate and lack documentation (ibid). Older men's ability to set up in business is often curtailed by age-related discrimination on the part of credit providers. Despite this, older men are often still financially responsible for younger family members. In both South Africa and Bangladesh, old age was defined by older men in HAI research as increasing dependency on others, due to physical limitations (such as loss of eyesight), declining mobility, and failing health, all of which make it difficult for them to contribute economically (HAI/BAAIGM et al 2000; Mohatle and Agyarko 1999). All HAI's studies reveal that older men experience feelings of rejection when they are no longer able to earn income.

In addition, older men do not seem to be as adaptable to changing situations as women. An interesting aspect of HAI's Ghana study is its analysis of the collapse of the mono-crop, cocoa, and the traumatising effect that this has had on older men. Older men still see a revitalised cocoa industry as the way out of their economic plight, while older women are busily making headway in agriculture and petty trading (Ahenkora 1999). In the 1990s in the Russian Federation, rapid social and economic change, community breakdown, and financial insecurity, including declining pension payments, have triggered alcoholism among many older men. Male life-expectancy fell from 65 to 58 between 1987 and 1994 (Gorman 1999).

Ironically, while older women's economic contributions are often underrated, by themselves and their community and family, they are accepted as retaining a useful role for longer than men, in that they are able and willing to continue reproductive work in the household, which is essential for family survival. Older men have difficulty in shifting their activities to these functional, household roles, owing to stigma, lack of confidence, or cultural barriers associated with performing 'women's work'. Those who do make the adjustment may be rewarded with care and prestige, as is the case in communities where elderly men are left to care for orphans whose parents have died of AIDS (Gurmessa 1999).

Older men are more likely to live with a spouse when they reach old age, due to women's longer life-expectancy in most regions and the accepted social practice of older men marrying younger women. However, when they are frail, the care they receive may not be appropriate, and there is little research in developing countries to explore this question. Chronic conditions linked to the natural ageing process, such as incontinence and dementia, may precipitate the abandonment and abuse of men. Research in St Lucia points out that more older men beg for a living than older women, and that they are less likely to be supported by their offspring than older women (HAI 2000, forthcoming).

Some research suggests that the tendency of men of all ages not to develop support structures among friends and community, as women do, results in greater exclusion of older men than women (Sheldon and Van Ommeren 1999).

Development responses to age and exclusion

Most international development programmes fail to support older women and men as they make their substantial economic and social contributions. Indeed, policy-makers are often unaware that older people – particularly women – make a contribution at all. This lack of basic knowledge leads to flawed policy-making.

Our experience is that it is rare for older people to be included in any discussion about issues that affect them directly. A widow aged 71, invited to an HAI research meeting in Bangladesh, stated: *'This is the first time I have been in a meeting like this. I want to do it again'* (HAI research report 1999, unpublished). This is a refrain that we commonly hear in HelpAge International. There is a tendency among policy-makers, development workers, younger people – and often some older people themselves – to assume that older people can have their concerns met through some form of welfare service. However, this is often very far from the needs and wishes of older people themselves. As an older Rwandan woman said to us during research on older people in emergencies: *'Why don't the agencies support our projects? This would be much better than us waiting for them to bring things to us. We want our projects to keep moving and growing – we can look after ourselves'* (HAI/UNHCR/ECHO 1999, 40).

How should support be offered? In the analysis of women's and men's experience of old age given above, it is clear that older people experience social and economic exclusion in the areas of health and material security/social status. Tensions between generations may result in violence and abuse, and violation of their human rights.

Health

Declining health and chronic impoverishment are huge barriers that daily confront older women and men in their struggle to survive and fulfil their obligations. The exclusion and powerlessness associated with ageing affect both women's and men's ability to interact with service providers, officials, and family members on key questions regarding welfare entitlements and care issues. For example, the principle of State provision of essential drugs for older people is meaningless if older people cannot reach health centres. Even if they do manage to get there, many older people are simply misdiagnosed or not treated, and simple, cheap, and effective operations, such as cataract removal to restore sight, are not routinely done. Gender-based discrimination means that women in particular have great difficulties in accessing and paying for modern medical care; older men tend not to seek medical help until there is a crisis. Older people the world over are likely to rely more than younger people on traditional remedies; although these may be expensive and are not always effective, they have the advantage of being accessible and can be paid for in kind, when resources are available (Ahenkora 1999).

Material security and social status

Some of the barriers preventing older women and men producers from accessing income are outlined in earlier sections. In countries that provide old-age pensions, this is often the most important source of income for older men and women. In some contexts, including South Africa, the pension is increasingly the economic mainstay of the entire family (Mohatle and Agyarko 1999). In such cases, the economic support to the extended family given by the pension raises the self-esteem and status of pension-holders as providers to the family. South African respondents told us: *'We are important to our families when we get our pensions.'* However, others told us that the pension can *'expose older persons to abuse by unscrupulous and uncaring family members'* (ibid).

Tensions between generations

The quotations above illustrate how chronic poverty and socio-economic change is placing increasing pressures on traditional family-based reciprocity. As a young woman interviewed in HAI's Lao study pointed out, poverty is the critical problem. *'Sometimes we have to care for our in-laws as well as our parents. Taking care of much older parents is very difficult – harder because we are very poor and do not have enough food'* (Graham 2000, 22).

Demographic change increases strains on hard-pressed family-support structures, as falling fertility rates combine with increasing longevity. The impact of phenomena such as HIV/AIDS, conflict-induced migration, and refugee resettlement has changed the expectations and behaviour of older and younger people. Rapid urbanisation and migration for work have begun significantly to alter family and community relationships. Urban living, with its restrictions on physical space, makes the close proximity of a relatively large number of family members of different generations more problematic.

Older people have to cope with changes in social status and changing attitudes to older men (and women in some cultures), who were often regarded in the past as a source of wisdom and knowledge. A common complaint in the Tanzania research was that, these days, older people had 'less support from the family and the community' (Forrester 1999, 60). But it has to be recognised that responsibility for the care of older people is falling on fewer children, and the impact is felt most by those with least resources.

These changes require flexibility and adaptation of older people, whose expectations of what would happen in old age may be turned upside down by forces beyond their control. Adaptation through training is hindered by high rates of illiteracy; the general lack of attention to the importance of education for older people is a further factor compounding exclusion and discrimination.

Violence and abuse

The nature and extent of the violence and abuse of older people by younger generations is only just becoming known. Abuse of older women by older men, reflecting a lifetime of gender inequality, is also being recorded. Older survivors of abuse are reluctant to come forward, because much of the abuse happens within the domestic environment, and they are both ashamed and afraid to disclose evidence (personal communication, 1999). Spurred on by the extreme example of witchcraft-related atrocities, social policy makers are only just beginning to track how abuse and violence is often linked to declining status and the barriers encountered in contributing to family survival. Abuse may take a number of forms. Physical abuse may include not only injury but also malnutrition or the withholding of physical care. Psychological abuse, such as threats, verbal assault, or isolation, may be used even where physical violence is absent. Indeed, in Chile, attitudes among the younger public and policy-makers that exclude older people and contribute to their vulnerability are considered to be a form of abuse (Lowick and Avalos 1999, 22).

Denial of basic human rights

In 1982, the Vienna Plan of Action on Ageing set specific targets for the inclusion of older people in social and economic development, and progress will be considered in the follow-up conference recently agreed for 2002 in Spain. The United Nations Social Summit of 1995 agreed an overarching priority to achieve 'a society for all', and affirmed that economic development, social development, and environmental protection for all people are interdependent and mutually reinforcing components of sustainable development. The most positive trend – and accompanying challenge – during the 1990s was the progressive recognition, by all ratifying governments, of the 1986 United Nations Declaration on the Right to Development for all people, regardless of age, gender, religion, class, nationality, and ethnic groupings. The 1999 report of the High Commissioner for Human Rights centred its argument on the importance of governments working to make measurable progress on recognising this right. The Beijing Declaration (UN 1995) provided an opportunity for older women, by urging an approach to development that was explicitly inclusive of women of all ages (paras 8, 32, 34).

However, the poverty of older women and men is still not included as a core concern in the social, economic, and ethical debates of our time. The 1999 report of the United Nations High Commissioner for Human Rights (UN 1999) did not mention age-based poverty, or the vulnerabilities of older women and men; likewise, age-related issues struggle for room in the current preparations for the historic Millennium Summit of the United Nations, in September 2000.

The way forward

A first step would be to recognise the rights of older people. HelpAge International is asking that the rights and contributions of older women and men be specifically acknowledged in the agreements of United

Nations conferences of recent years. We are also suggesting that the specific rights of older people be developed into a legal charter to form part of the body of international rights-based agreements, drawing on the key 'Principles' for Older Persons mentioned at the start of this article, in UN Resolution 46/91.

Older people's immense contribution to social and economic development needs to be acknowledged. The key policy question facing development policy-makers today is not *what should we do about older people?,* but *what would the rest of us do without them?* Both socially and economically, can we really afford to ignore their contributions any longer? Policy-makers must recognise that investment in the productive and social capacities of older women and men is likely to yield far-reaching results in terms of community welfare and economic return.

In general, basic research with and about older people needs much improvement. As this article has shown, research that involves the participation of older people themselves reveals quite different realities from those assumed hitherto by policy-makers. In particular, the views and needs of older women need to be taken into account in research or policy in a systematic way. For example, HAI research has revealed that, while all older persons fare very badly in emergencies, older women's cultural, social, and health needs are often blatantly ignored – despite the critical role that they can and do play in keeping fragmented families together, and in rebuilding lives in the aftermath of crisis. Research and action on age-sensitive and gender-sensitive health and nutrition issues, the needs of older people, and appropriate strategies to deal with them are deficient everywhere, particularly in the developing world (Peachey 1999).

Older people doing development

Analysis and planning for development programmes should involve older people themselves. Sensitivity to gender, culture, language, and tradition must be built in to this work. HAI is supporting a portfolio of projects throughout the world to enable impoverished older women and men, who often have little formal education, to become successful community-based gerontologists, educators, para-legal workers, teachers, nutritionists, organisers of full-scale emergency-relief programmes, and community activists.

It makes economic sense, as well as being good development, to invest in schemes run and managed by older people – and HAI is collecting data to show this. For example, HAI research in Juba, southern Sudan, has shown that community work targeting older people in this region of armed conflict has enabled relief aid to be targeted very effectively. The distribution of essential non-food items was an incentive for older people to come together and begin a dialogue between them and partner non-government organisations (NGOs). The participation of older people in the relief programme supported their empowerment, as the programme scaled up to reach over 2000 more people than originally envisaged, and older people themselves managed major elements of this work, including brick manufacture, the construction of houses and pit-latrines, and the management of committees. Awareness was raised about the abilities, rights, and capacities of older people across all sectors of civil society and government. The programme has now evolved from an emergency intervention to a more sustainable development process, which has older people at its centre (*Ageways*, October 1999).

In general, greater numbers of older women tend to be involved in HAI's project work than older men, although men can and do become involved. For example, a Council of Venerable Old Persons has been formed in Bolivia from a group of male beggars who organised themselves to demand legal documentation; the council has female and male members now. Male and female authority conferred by conventional assumptions about gender relations, as well as long life and experience, can and should be used in humanitarian and development work.

In advocacy for change, HAI's experience is that change more readily comes about when older people organise into groups to make their own voices heard. In Latin America and the Caribbean, such organisation has led to significant advances at both grassroots and policy-making levels of society. Older people have pioneered approaches to such diverse activities as legal documentation, prevention of elder abuse, national policy-formulation, and care standards in hospitals and old people's homes.

Conclusion

The key to change is to re-orientate development and social policy, so that they value and support the contributions of older women and men to their families and communities, while also seeking out and responding to their age- and gender-based needs and predicaments. It is more imperative than ever that we heed the 1995 Copenhagen Declaration that 'generations need to invest in one another and recognise diversity and generational interdependence, guided by the twin principles of reciprocity and equity' (UNIS 1995). This is not to deny the rights of other vulnerable groups, but to seek inclusion of a critical part of the world's population that is consistently left out of the picture.

Sylvia Beales is Policy Development Manager at HelpAge International, 67–74 Saffron Hill, London EC1N 8QX, UK. Hai@helpage.org; www.helpage.org

Notes

1 Red eyes are caused by a lifetime of cooking over smoky fires.

References

Ageways, No. 52, October 1999, HelpAge International, UK

Ahenkora, K (1999), *The Contributions of Older People to Development, the Ghana Study*, HelpAge International and HelpAge Ghana, available from HAI

Lowick J and Avalos R (1999), *Maltrato en la Vejez, Orientaciones Generales para su Investigacion* Centro de Capacitacion (CEC) Study Document 1, Chile

De Haan, A (1998), 'Social exclusion: an alternative concept for the study of deprivation?', *IDS Bulletin*, Vol. 20, No.1, Institute of Development Studies, University of Sussex, UK

Forrester, K (1999), *The Situation of Older People in Tanzania*, HelpAge International (research report available from HAI)

Gorman, M (1999), 'The situation of older people in the transitional economies of Eastern and Central Europe' in *The Ageing and Development Report*, HelpAge International and Earthscan,UK

Graham, J (2000), *Understanding the Situation of Older People in the Laos PDR: participatory rural appraisal of older people*, Government of Laos Department of Labour and Social Welfare, and HelpAge International, (publication forthcoming, available from HAI)

Gurmessa M (1999), 'Social Effects of Aids on the Elderly', unpublished report, Ethiopia

HAI (HelpAge International) (forthcoming), *Care of the Elderly in St Lucia*, HAI for the Government of St. Lucia (available from HAI)

HAI/Earthscan (1999), *The Ageing and Development Report*, HelpAge International and Earthscan, UK

HAI/BAAIGM/BRAC/RIC/BWHC (HAI with the Bangladesh Association for the Aged and Institute for Geriatric Medicine, Bangladesh Rural Advancement Committee, Resource Integration Centre, and Bangladesh Women's Health Coalition) (2000), 'A Situation Analysis of Older People in Bangladesh – "Uncertainty rules our lives"', unpublished report

HAI/UNHCR/ECHO (HAI with United Nations High Commission for Refugees, and the European Community Humanitarian Office (1999), *The Ageing World and Humanitarian Crisis: Background Research Papers*, UK

HAI/UNHCR/ECHO (2000), *Older People in Disasters and Humanitarian Crises: Guidelines for Best Practice*, UK

Heslop, A (1999), *Ageing and Development*, DFID Working Paper No.3, DFID,UK

Lowick, J and Avalos, R (1999), *Maltrato en la Vejez, Orientaciones Generales para su Investigacion*, Centro de Capacitacion (CEC), Study Document 1, Chile

Mohatle, T and Agyarko, de G (1999), *The Contributions of Older People to Development, the South Africa Study*, HelpAge International, UK

Owen, M (1999), *A World of Widows*, Zed Press, UK

Peachey, K (1999), *Ageism – A Factor in the Nutritional Vulnerability of Older People* HAI/ODI (report available from HAI)

Sheldon, T and Van Ommeren, T (1999), *Portraits of Ageing Women*, Wemos Foundation, Amsterdam, The Netherlands

Sim, C-S and Ree, K-O (1997), 'Variations in preferred living arrangements among Korean elderly parents' in *Journal of Cross Cultural Gerontology*, Vol. 12, No. 2

UN (1995), *Beijing Platform of Action*, UN, USA

UN (1996), *Sex and Age Quinquennial 1950–2050*, UN, USA

UN (1999), Report of the High Commissioner for Human Rights, Agenda Item 14(h), delivered at the Substantive Session of 1999, 5-30 July 1999

UNIS (United Nations Information Service) (1995), Report of World Summit for Development, Copenhagen, New York/Geneva

UNFPA (United Nations Population Fund) (1998), *State of the World Population*, UN, USA

UNFPA and CGBS (Population and Family Study Centre) (1999), *Population Ageing: Challenges for policies and programmes in developed and developing countries*, UNFPA and CBGS, Belgium

WHO (World Health Organisation) (1999), *Ageing: Exploding the myths*, Ageing and Health

'At my age I should be sitting under that tree':
the impact of AIDS on Tanzanian lakeshore communities

Judith Appleton

In 1992, the author led a participatory rural appraisal (PRA) exercise for a community fisheries project in Kagera region, on the western side of Lake Victoria, Tanzania. The PRA team visited four settlements: the prime harbour settlement on Kerebe Island; N'toro beach, in Bukoba district, near the Ugandan border; Chamkwikwi landing site in Muleba district; and Buzirayombo bay settlement in Biharamulo district in the south. This article draws on that research, to give an outsider's analysis of the ways in which AIDS was changing livelihoods in poor fishing and farming communities.[1] On the lakeshore and islands, adults were falling ill and dying. This loss of men and women in their prime was causing major economic and social stresses for the single parents, grandparents, and orphans whom we met. They showed resilience and adaptability in the face of this threat to their already precarious livelihoods. The article ends by suggesting ways in which development policy makers and practitioners should support livelihoods in the era of AIDS.

Lake Victoria has long supported an artisanal fishing industry, and fish-processing and marketing activities which extend far beyond its shores. Throughout East Africa, the work of catching, drying, selling, and transporting the small *dagaa* (L. *rastrineobola argentea*) provides a variety of ways of making an income. Ultimately, the *dagaa* ensures a tasty relish for eating with maize-meal, or *nsima*. Along the way, it provides a means of support to many: the lakeshore farmers who share-crew on the boats (similar to share-cropping on land); the women who are involved in processing the fish and gathering grass for the drying-beds; the general and specialised traders; the casual labourers; and all kinds of large- and small-scale entrepreneurs along the supply chain. Other native species of fish, including *haplochromis* and *tilapia*, are sun-dried or smoked on wood or grass, and have also been part of the lake's fish trade.

Around 1970, the giant Nile perch found its way to Lake Victoria from the lakes in the north, where it had first been introduced in the 1960s. It spread to all parts of Lake Victoria, except the shallow

bays. Twenty-five years later, this carnivorous, deep-dwelling species not only dominated the catch of fish in the lake, but had also consumed most of the other species (including *haplochromis, cichlids,* and *tilapia*) in the depths of the shallow lake. However, it has not affected the *dagaa*, which are a surface species.

Livelihoods in Kagera

The appearance of the giant perch may have been a disaster for all those palates – local and farther afield – that were fond of the succulent though bony *cichlids* and *tilapia*; but it was a boon to poor Haya cash-croppers.

Haya people were originally pastoralists, who were living in this area prior to colonisation in the mid-nineteenth century. The colonial regime introduced coffee cultivation to Bukoba and Muleba, in the hilly north, and cotton in the flatter, hotter southern part of Muleba. Haya men became cash-croppers, relying on their wives to produce the maize and banana staples for the family. At first, they were little involved in the fisheries, which were small-scale and a minority occupation before the advent of the Nile perch. Subsequently, the money to be earned from the growing perch-fishing activity led them to turn their hand to this developing industry, which relied on many related occupations from boat building and gear production, through fish-processing, to trade. The incomes gained from these activities sustained lakeshore families and, in addition, provided money for small-scale investment in agricultural activities. The economic viability of this livelihood, combining fishing and agricultural activities, relies on adult men taking the main role in boat-fishing, and adult women taking responsibility for farming.

In 1992, at the time of the PRA exercise on which this article is based, most lakeshore fishermen (and even most boat-owners) to whom we spoke regarded their farms as the family's mainstay. They went fishing when they were not needed for heavy work on the farm, and used their pay to buy clothes for the family, or agricultural equipment. The fish they kept were used for the family pot, or given to fellow villagers, to cement friendly relations. The exceptions, who lived exclusively on their labour from fishing, were single men, most at the prime harbour settlement of Kerebe Island.

At the time of the research, the average size of the Nile perch being caught in Lake Victoria was declining. This indicated a decrease in perch population. Another sign was the resurgence of the *cichlids* and other species, which was already being welcomed by local people: these fish are preferred to the oily and relatively tasteless perch, and their reappearance restored culinary variety. However, the decrease in the perch population was a potential threat to livelihoods: not only to the profits from perch-fishing, processing (smoking and salting), and legal and illegal trading, but to feeder occupations. Disaster loomed over the majority of lake-fishers, who depended on the industry to supplement their farming incomes.

Meanwhile, the makings of another disaster – that of AIDS – were already present in the area. Eight years on, there are one million AIDS cases in Tanzania, and 940,000 people have already died. Since the beginning of the epidemic, 730,000 children have lost both their parents to AIDS (Hivinsite, 12 May 2000).

Factors contributing to HIV infection

In addition to the fisheries boom-and-bust culture, there were other significant structural and institutional factors contributing to a high prevalence of HIV infection in Kagera. (It should be pointed out that in PRA sessions, people mentioned various factors in addition to the economic and social factors mentioned below. There were rumours in Kagera that suggested a wish to explain the AIDS epidemic as an outside influence: for example, that medical blood supplies came from the army and the prisons, where no HIV/AIDS screening was carried out.)

A key factor is the pattern of temporary migration of male fishers to settlements by the lake. Since perch-fishing began, temporary fishing camps of grass huts and sheds have grown up seasonally on the lakeshore, with predominantly male populations. Male labour relies, for food, drink and sexual services, on cafés, tea-shops, and bars, largely run by women. Each camp is associated with particular farming communities, which may be at a distance of up to 15 kilometres from the shore. Some of the population of the camps – particularly on the islands in the lake – consists of migrant and casual labourers from farther away. The potential for the spread of HIV infection is obvious.

Kagera borders Uganda's Rakai province, where HIV prevalence among young working adults in trading centres and rural areas was found to be high in 1989: 43 per cent among men in their twenties, and 52 per cent among women of the same age-group (Barnett and Blaikie 1992, 32). In Rakai, the Ganda people's patterns of frequent and diverse sexual relationships, including transient ones, have been a widely acknowledged factor in the rapid spread of HIV infection. A similar pattern of sexual behaviour is a feature of the lives of Kagera's Haya population. A Haya woman traditionally occupies an inferior position in the household. Until the middle of the twentieth century, her subservience was rendered visible in the heavy metal ankle rings that restricted her mobility. Traditionally, she was secluded for eight months after marriage, and fed a restricted non-protein diet, allegedly to control her sexuality as well as to teach her generally to mind her place in the family and society. That place included accepting social, economic, and legal dependence, polygamy, and marital violence, and showing deference to the men in the household. A Haya man might divorce a wife for many reasons, including lack of a male heir, adultery, or sexually transmitted disease (Pratt, personal communication).

Together with growing food crops (while her husband tended the livestock, and later grew cash-crops and fished), the bearing of children was a Haya woman's main role in marriage. However, these children might be the fruit of unions with other men within her husband's family or with friends, instigated by her husband or his relatives, rather than her own idea, which would have been cause for divorce. Fathers-in-law had rights to sexual relations with their sons' new wives on the first night of marriage, and there was a common practice of wife-sharing with other male relatives of the husband, and as hospitality to the household's male visitors. The children might even be claimed by the biological fathers according to *bisisi* – the right of first intercourse after menstruation or a birth. Before marriage, a Haya girl might have sexual experience deriving from this rule of hospitality, but pre-marital pregnancy was not tolerated. Consequently, Haya girls have been married off young, to prevent them being drowned or ostracised should they become pregnant before marriage. As recently as the 1950s, early marriage was also a defence against girls being taken to be concubines to the 'royal' lineages (Pratt, personal communication)

In the 1920s and 1930s, significant numbers of Haya women found a way to escape daily drudgery and their subjugation to husbands and chiefs. While some girls and women found havens in Christian missions, others turned their experience of sex with different partners, born of subservience in marriage, to economic benefit. Making use of the new road, steamer, and rail links to travel, Haya women became known as among the more desirable, and best organised, commercial sex workers in urban areas throughout East Africa. A contributory factor to the enterprise of prostitution may well have been a spirit-medium movement (*embandwa*), which has not completely disappeared among Haya women, and provided a focus for their resistance to male and royal control of their behaviour and fertility, exempted them from field-work, and freed them to travel, to dance, and to charge fees for their services (Pratt, personal communication)

The PRA revealed that gender relations have changed significantly since then: material, social, and economic developments have increased Haya women's opportunities to determine their own lives, and have transformed many traditional relationships. Haya woman may now divorce their husbands, and these days the majority of women-instigated divorces are on grounds of husbands' neglect or inability to support the household. However, much still survives: not least, the sexual legacy. Many Haya women are still commercial sex workers; some have earned enough to support their families back home and buy their own land. Participants in the PRA told us that other former sex workers have returned to Kagera and appear to have avoided AIDS; they are heading their own households, and frequently rank among the better-off in the community.

The impact of AIDS on livelihoods in Kagera

The next section moves beyond a health-related focus on sexual behaviour and HIV transmission to examine the impact of AIDS-related illness and death on the livelihoods of fisher–farmer households. In particular, it considers the impact of the deaths of young and middle-aged adults of both sexes on the economic survival of household members, who are predominantly elderly people and children.

Overall, the impact of AIDS illness and death on livelihoods in Kagera is in many respects similar to that in other rural settings of sub-Saharan Africa. The loss of adults in the prime of life leads to serious labour shortages for fishing and farming, in addition to child-care and household maintenance. The symbiosis between male-dominated fishing and female-dominated farming, on which household survival depends, ceases if adults of either sex fall ill or die. More dependants rely on a smaller number of productive family members. The decline in the productive (and reproductive) capacity of the household leads to a loss of fishery income, a knock-on loss of investment in the farm and / or reduced agricultural production, and changes to agricultural decisions because of a need to save labour (for example, which crops to grow, or whether to leave land fallow). This in turn leads to a general decline in household income and access to food. This needs to be made up by the sale of fishing or farming equipment (in turn constraining the remaining productive activities), by sale of other assets, and by the spending of savings, and/or remittances from absent fishermen, on household survival. The need to care for anyone with AIDS-related illnesses leads to an increase in household expenditure on medical treatment, transport, and special foods.

This cycle not only spells a descent into deeper poverty throughout the region, but is further exacerbated by the social and economic stigma experienced by relatives of people known to have AIDS. The issue of stigma came up in the PRA that we carried out in Biharamulo. The fact that Biharamulo is the one district out of the four that we visited with a lower Haya population may suggest there is less stigma attached to AIDS in Haya villages.

Direct costs

Women in the villages to which N'toro fishermen belong told us that the costs of care during illness were minimal, since *'There are no medicines … well, the clinic's closed. The sick ones are just weak, have no appetite and sit around indoors. And the men don't bring in money or fish. That's much worse.'* The women were far freer with their comments than the men, some of whom were now single parents. One woman said: *'A husband with AIDS is worse than a lazy husband, because you can't divorce him – it's not his fault.'* Women we met at the clinic in Biharamulo claimed that there were medical costs, but could not specify how much.

Food security and diets

The local porridge (*matoke*) is made of plantain and beans: it contained relatively fewer beans in the poorer households we visited, and these families also eat fish infrequently. The effect on a family's food of a combination of reduced income, labour-saving cropping, and limited access to fish, is clearly poorer diets. Poor diets in turn reduce resistance to any infection.

One woman in Muleba told us that she had a friend caring for a sick brother, who was being advised by a clinic supported by a foreign HIV/AIDS project to buy and prepare food for him that she could not afford for her children. Her friends thought she should feed the children better instead.

Changes in the inter-generational division of labour

There were striking differences in the composition of the fisher populations in the camps on Kerebe Island, and those in the village and on the beach at N'toro, the northernmost camp we visited. In Kerebe harbour, the 'boom-town' of perch-fishing, the beach was crowded with energetic fishermen. Their usual behaviour was to leap out of their boats, grab their pay, and make straight for the *pombe* (banana home-brew) bars until the next day. Because Kerebe is the most lucrative place to fish and to offer fishing labour, there is a constant flow of young male labourers through the harbour town of Furuza, some of whom have left wives or parents to take care of children and farms on the lakeshore.

On Kerebe, there are few children, social structures are undeveloped, and there is no police force. However, the island – and the settlement of Furuza in particular – is run like a feudal realm, controlled by four 'perch lords' and their retainers. The perch lords have offices on the hillsides overlooking the harbour, where they own bars as well as boats and equipment enterprises. We were told in PRA sessions that labour laws were brushed aside here: the perch lords hire and fire at will, profiting both from the abundant catches in the middle of the lake, and from the low wages that they are able to pay. Few labourers actually complain, because of the widespread desperation that drives people out here to subsist for a season. Some are even persuaded to take part in the illegal export trade to Uganda of the prized perch

bladders, in boats that make the run under cover of night to evade the coastguards.

By contrast, in lakeshore N'toro, there were children with their fathers and brothers on the beach, watching the landings and helping to hold the nets during mending. There were also several quite elderly men who were not just mending nets (a usual activity for older men) but also crewing and engaged in beach-seining (shore-based fishing)

Case study 1: a grandparent-headed household

One of the elderly men on the shore at N'toro took us to meet his equally elderly wife, who was making reed mats in a shelter along the beach, while looking after three grandchildren, including a toddler. Their son and daughter-in-law had died recently of AIDS. The grandparents were doing full-time child-care: she provided the secure base, while he kept the older ones amused and busy. They had found it impossible to replace the labour of their son and daughter-in-law in the boat and on the farm, since the old man was not sprightly and the old woman had a bad leg. *'I should be sitting under that tree at my age, not working in the sun,'* said the old man. *'All this will drive me to an early grave, but not as early as my son, I guess.'*

The solution for the extended family had been for the grandparents to move in with a daughter, in the same village. They had enlarged her house, and with the money that the old man made from the fishing and the old woman earned from her mats their daughter was able to hire labour to maintain both her own land and half that belonging formerly to the dead son and daughter-in-law. She was able to provide all of them with maize and plantains. The village chief's spokesman told us that the old couple had been allowed to use their son's land after his death, since the village had plenty of land. He said the problem for the elders was to make sure that enough land was being cultivated to feed everyone, particularly in that year when cash-crop (coffee) prices were low. This way of living was just adequate to ensure the extended family's survival until the next death, or until the old man or woman was unable to continue to work.

Case study 2: a child-headed household

On N'toro beach we also met a household consisting of orphan boys, the eldest of whom was 14. They had chosen to live on their own. The village chief's spokesman told us that orphans were generally taken in by relatives or neighbours, but there were more and more of them, and he did not know how families would cope if it continued, even though orphaned children could offer their labour for farming.

The orphaned teenager household-head had been taken on in his dead father's place in the 'best' boat in N'toro (the only one whose owner had acquired an engine for it). The boy was delighted to have been taken on, although he was only getting half-pay, and he had to wrestle with the other crew for his share of the landed catch. The boat-owner would not talk to us. The older man mentioned in the case study above commented that the boat-owner had been reluctant to take on the boy, since he wanted experienced men in the boat now that it was powered to take them farther out on the lake, but he had bowed to community pressure. He commented that the boy was one of many who were desperate to work and, since the boat-owner had to finance his engine, it was not surprising that he wasn't giving money away in higher wages.

The local jobbing fishermen had taken their own initiative vis-à-vis the gang of younger boys on the beach who had lost fathers and needed fish for their suppers. They had worked out a formula to incorporate them into the work of beach-seining and to share the catch with them. The men rowed one end of the net out from the shore, dropped it, and rowed back, pulling the end into an arc against the current, while the beach team on the other end was composed of a line-up of adults and children, in order of decreasing size. The youngest involved were around ten years old. As the net came in, the larger fish were picked out and went to the men, while the boys got smaller ones, according to both their stature and the contribution they had made to pulling the net in. The formula was working: there was little squabbling.

Women, widowhood, and changes in the gender division of labour

Many changes in the gendered division of labour are likely when Haya women are widowed and take on household headship. Colonial legislation of 1944 has acquired a new importance in the context of men's deaths from AIDS. This legislation recognised Haya women's right to inherit their husbands' farmland. At the time it was passed, the legislation was likely to have been a measure intended to forestall destitution among women who were losing access to land, since this was being increasingly occupied by men for use as coffee plantations (Pratt, personal communication).

In contrast, non-Haya women from Mwanza, whom we met on Kerebe Island, told us of the emotional distress and economic destitution caused by their in-laws claiming the estate of the women's deceased husbands – including the children, as well as land and material possessions. We noted that non-Haya women were now working in other parts of the fisheries industry: for example, Kerebe Island boasted a fish-smoking enterprise owned and run by women. Haya women are restricted to selected parts of fish-processing, reflecting the strict gender division of labour of their pastoralist past, when men cared for the livestock and women were restricted to milking.

From our observations, fish-cleaning for smoking, and the smoking itself, is men's work.

On Kerebe, a female boat-owner (a non-Haya divorcée based in Mwanza) commented that, for Haya women, *'trade and industry are not really their sort of thing'*. Her suggestion that Haya women's investments were concentrated in land and in the tea-shop sector was borne out in all four sites we visited. On Kerebe, it was Haya women making a livelihood from sexual exchange: fishermen in the bar that some of the PRA team patronised told them that there was a brisk demand for Haya 'wives', contracted for the season. In Biharamulo, Haya divorcées returning from the sex industry in Dar es Salaam and elsewhere were also accused of bringing AIDS back with them, but this type of remark was not made to us in the more predominantly Haya districts of Muleba and Bukoba.

The female boat-owner mentioned above was visiting Kerebe to supervise the hiring of labour and the negotiations over shares for the season for her boat's crew. She told us that it had been tough hanging on to assets from her marriage, but tougher still finding that she was excluded from much of the networking that goes on among the owners of boats: all the rest were male. She thought there were unlikely to be many widows entering the fishing industry at higher levels.

One sign of stress among women, as the communities face fish depletion and reduced productive capacity due to AIDS, was competition over fuel-grass, a common property resource, on the island of Kerebe. Wooded areas around Kagera are largely exhausted, and large quantities of grass are needed as a substitute underlay for drying the fish, and as fuel for smoking it. The job of grass collection is consigned to women, and the sale of grass as fuel provides important income. This job is becoming increasingly competitive, with ever-larger numbers of women turning to it to meet their subsistence needs. There are wide variations in the money to be made from the activity: in spring and summer, the price is low while grass is abundant; in autumn and winter, a higher price reflects scarcity. We witnessed tussles going on between the perch lords' retainers, who were setting fire to the grasslands to generate better growth, and women desperately trying to smother the fires and cut the grass before it caught fire.

Shoreline work on *dagaa* fish-drying is limited to a maximum of ten days a month, since fishing *dagaa* takes place only during the dark quarter of the moon. This work consists of grass-cutting and supply, by women, and the spreading, turning, and collecting of the fish, by men. The only exception to this division of labour that we encountered was in a family enterprise on Kerebe Island, where a woman was helping her sick husband with the turning and collecting. She told us that this would maximise earnings from the catch as long as he was well enough to go out fishing, but that she would subsequently have to find cash to buy fish for her family.

Does AIDS herald 'de-development'?

AIDS is a tragedy for the individual men, women, and children who are directly and indirectly affected by it, and presents a threat to the livelihoods of households, communities, and – ultimately – whole countries.

In Kagera, as in communities throughout sub-Saharan Africa, women and men, old and young, are adapting their way of life to enable them to cope with the impact of the illness and deaths of adults in their most productive years. In Kagera, we witnessed people coping in various ways. Adaptations that we judged to have a negative impact in the longer term are summarised as follows:

- land falling fallow and into disuse as a result of AIDS-related shortages of household labour;
- children taken out of school because parents can no longer afford the fees, due to adult illness and death in the family;
- increasing numbers of children working (although we did not come across this, the potential for the unscrupulous to exploit children's and whole families' desperation is there);
- downward pressure on fishing wages, as casual work is sought by members of AIDS-depleted families, and a buyer's market develops;
- lower-value diets in families adapting to loss of income, food crops, and fish;
- increasingly regular income from commercial sex work (commonly through tea-houses and *pombe* bars), particularly for women who lack other skills, or who decide that this is the easiest way to earn cash for children's upkeep.

Positive ways of coping with the impact of AIDS-related illness and death also existed in Kagera. We judged these to include:

- villagers taking in orphaned children who were not relatives, leading to their being able to maintain food production with the extra labour (we witnessed this occurring in cases where children had already given up school, and others where they had left when school fees could no longer be paid);
- conscious adaptation of lake- and, particularly, beach-fishing, to enable AIDS orphans to participate and feed themselves;
- other methods of coping at community levels, including pragmatic land-use arrangements designed to help the needy families, which effectively change patterns of tenure.

We also noted various socio-cultural phenomena and anomalies related to HIV and AIDS. The first two of these concern transmission of HIV. First, there are mixed messages about the safety of breast-feeding in communities where there are high levels of HIV infection and no testing is available. Breast-milk supplies high levels of immunity to infection, and current international guidelines (WHO, 15 May 2000) recommend breast-feeding, particularly in contexts such as Kagera where there is no safe alternative, and where most infants are at high risk of morbidity and mortality from diarrhoeal disease and other infections, especially if they are bottle-fed. However, at the time we visited the area, at least one international NGO working in the area was counselling against breast-feeding by HIV-positive mothers. Secondly, we noted the phenomenon of noisy, new Christian youth groups, whose members are asked to pledge themselves in public to sexual abstinence before marriage, and monogamy within it: a source of some amusement to the staff in our hotel, where we were regularly entertained by different groups.

Another set of social phenomena affects those living with HIV and AIDS. Around Kagera, fishermen who know they have the virus have joined outlaw groups on the islands, providing the cheap labour on which whole communities – such as that run on Kerebe by the perch lords – are built. They are believed, probably correctly, by the surrounding community to be spreading the disease. In these communities, there is widespread alcoholism, particularly featuring *pombe* and distilled banana alcohol.

What is needed for the future?

Development organisations working in regions affected by a high prevalence of HIV/AIDS need urgently to develop their understanding of the economic and social processes triggered by this disease (Barnett and Blaikie 1992). It kills those of productive age, and leaves children and elderly people to make a livelihood as best they can. This suggests additional development priorities in the supporting of livelihoods of AIDS-depleted households. HIV/AIDS is not only a health issue that demands prevention and care for the sick; it is also a livelihoods issue, since, if AIDS-depleted households are not the target of particular support, the precarious livelihoods of survivors are likely to collapse under the impact of the epidemic.

Our PRA exercises enabled us to make a tentative and preliminary exploration of the impact of AIDS in Kagera. There is now an urgent need for case studies like this to be followed up and verified, for pointers given here to emerging trends and coping strategies to be amplified, and for lessons to be drawn from them and applied. Rapid research, identifying livelihood trends in AIDS-affected areas, should lead to establishing the validity, extent, and development of the above trends and others, the setting of precise targeting criteria for household vulnerability due to AIDS-depletion, and the provision of precise and appropriate support packages for different types of household.

Government, funding agencies, and NGOs involved in development need to adopt a consultative approach, to identify the key occupations that need support in local AIDS-depleted populations. This will allow invention and adaptation to flourish, as it did in the case of the N'toro fishermen's own initiative to ensure that AIDS orphans were able to take part in seine-fishing. In particular, because women generally have fewer social rights, for example to land, support is needed for those women's enterprises that help them and their families to survive despite AIDS illness and death in the household. This support would include promoting

women's access to credit, labour, inputs, and information. It is also important to combine these with support for education (for example, in-school feeding) to encourage continued school attendance by the children of AIDS-depleted families.

Judith Appleton is a food-security specialist. She was working for FAO's Fisheries Department when she visited Kagera. For her work as a nutritionist with Save The Children Fund(UK) during the 1983-85 famine in Ethiopia, the UK government made her an MBE (Member of the Order of the British Empire). Her address is 197 Knowlwood Road, Todmorden, West Yorkshire, OL14 6PF, UK. E-mail: judith.appleton@zen.co.uk

Note

1 The primary source of information for this article comes from the PRA exercise with members of Haya fishing communities in Kagera, and interviews with key informants. The article is based on more women's voices than men's, since I was involved in more of the women's interviews. The article also draws on subsequent discussions and communications with Marion Pratt, on her own findings in the course of anthropological research in the region.

References

Appleton J (1993), *Lake Victoria Fisheries and Development in Kagera Region, Tanzania*, report for GCP/INT/467/NOR to URT/90/005, FAO Rome

Barnett A and Blaikie PM (1992), *AIDS in Africa: Its present and future impact*, The Guildford Press, London.

Hivinsite http://hivinsite.ucsf.edu/international/africa

WHO (World Health Organisation) http://www.who.int/chd/publication/newslet/dialog/9/update

Providing sex education to adolescents in rural Bangladesh:
experiences from BRAC

Sabina Faiz Rashid

The Bangladesh Rural Advancement Committee (BRAC) set up an Adolescent Reproductive Health Education (ARHE) programme in 1995, to provide information about reproductive health to adolescents in rural areas. New ideas and information are breaking the silence and shame about 'sensitive' topics, and proving a positive influence on the relationships between adolescents and their parents and teachers, and among adolescents themselves.

Twenty-three per cent of the total population of Bangladesh is aged between ten and 19. Over the next decade, these adolescents will enter their prime reproductive years. Like other South Asian states, Bangladesh is a conservative country. In addition to the effect of conservatism and strong patriarchal structures, rural Bangladesh is influenced by Islam, Hinduism, and traditional religious beliefs. The predominantly traditional and conservative nature of Bangladeshi society demands that young unmarried adolescent girls are modest and – at least in theory – sheltered from sexuality and knowledge of sexual reproduction. Low levels of education combine to create an environment of misunderstanding regarding reproductive and sexual health (Nahar, Amin et al, 1999).

Despite the fact that socio-cultural values in Bangladesh prohibit premarital sexual activity, research findings indicate that about half of all young men in rural areas have pre-marital sex, although the figures are lower for women, who are subject to greater social control (Aziz and Maloney 1985, cited in Caldwell and Pieris 1999). Moral disapproval of sexual activities outside marriage means that overall discussion and knowledge of such issues tend to be limited. Friends and older cousins, brothers, and sisters are the main source of information for adolescents, but these informants are often ignorant about reproductive health matters themselves. As a result, young adolescents have inadequate knowledge and often indulge in risky behaviour.

The ARHE programme

In 1995, the Bangladesh Rural Advancement Committee (BRAC)[1] set up an Adolescent Reproductive Health Education (ARHE) programme. ARHE classes are provided through BRAC's Basic Education for Older Children (BEOC) or Kishor Kishori (KK) schools, which run for three years. Pupils are adolescent boys and girls over the age of 12 who have never been enrolled in school. They are from very poor socio-economic backgrounds. Almost all parents are illiterate and have had very little formal schooling. ARHE classes are provided in the third year of schooling.

They are taught by women teachers who have primary education to Grade 9, from within the same community. ARHE education is also provided in BRAC's community libraries (*pathaghar*), and government secondary schools. Classes are taught for an hour a fortnight in the KK schools, and once a month in the community libraries (assessment report, 1999). Currently there are 803 institutions teaching ARHE, with approximately 27,175 students.

The current ARHE curriculum, introduced in 1998, includes education on the physical and mental changes experienced during adolescence; female and male physiology; and the process of reproduction, including conception, pregnancy, and childbearing, and guidance on the age at which marriage and childbearing should take place; sexually transmitted diseases; family planning and disease prevention; substance abuse, including smoking; and gender issues, including inequality between males and females, the need for respect between sexes, the role of males and females in reproduction, and violence against women and young girls.

The research

This article explores the effects of the ARHE programme on adolescent girls and boys, their parents, and community members; discusses the perceptions and concerns of adolescents as they face many psychological, social, and cultural changes; and explores the various factors influencing community acceptance of the programme. It draws on research into the impact of the programme in Nilphamari district, one of the first districts where the programme was set up. The field research was carried out from mid-October to the end of November 1999, in KK schools and community libraries. Research methods used included focus groups, participant observation, and semi-structured interviews with adolescents, mothers and aunts, teachers, and BRAC programme staff. The semi-structured interviews were carried out privately with individuals, to allow respondents to speak freely on taboo topics. Adolescent boys were interviewed by male researchers, and girls by female researchers. We cross-checked data to allow for exaggeration or bias in some of the adolescents' responses, and the numerous anecdotal stories told by many participants.

Findings

Community acceptance of the programme

The fact that the ARHE's classes have been held without any disruption from village members reveals a measure of acceptance of the programme so far. This may be partly because family-planning programmes targeting adults have already introduced the idea of family planning, and family-planning methods, into rural communities in Bangladesh (Mita and Simmons 1995). Like them, the ARHE programme is directing information on reproductive health knowledge at community level. Other factors that are likely to have led to this acceptance include the growing urbanisation of rural areas, the modernising influences of the electronic media, and increasing exposure to the views of NGOs, such as BRAC, which have been working in these areas for long periods of time.

Key issues for girls and boys

Adolescent girls reported that menstruation was the most significant topic discussed at the classes. In Bangladesh, this is associated with sexuality, fertility, and pollution, and is considered a shameful and hidden subject. Soon after the onset of menstruation, adolescent girls – particularly in rural areas – are married off (although this practice is changing in some regions – Rashid and Michaud 2000). The social taboos surrounding menstruation are so great that young adolescent girls and their mothers usually do not share their experiences and knowledge of menstruation. A recent research study carried out in both rural and urban areas of Bangladesh with adolescents aged between ten and 19 found that, out of 232 girls, only 34 per cent knew about menstruation before experiencing it, and as a result they found it mentally traumatic. After the onset of menstruation, many of these girls confided in their elder sisters, sisters-in-law, or grandmothers, who in turn gave them information on how to manage their menstruation. However, in most cases, the information given was incomplete (Nahar, Huq et al 1999).

Our research confirmed that the onset of menstruation can be a particularly traumatic time. One girl said: *'I had my menses when I was 12 years old ... I was really very scared. I thought I am dying. Blood was coming out. I went to my bhabi (sister-in-law), but she sent me to my older sister.'* A number of the girls said they were now using their new knowledge of hygienic menstruation practices gained through the ARHE, and discussing their new knowledge with other girls in the village. The diffusion of knowledge among girls took place informally, in after-school chats and in the community library. One girl explained: *'We usually sit and talk together with the other girls in the village. That is when they ask me about what I am learning in class. One girl came... and I told her what I know – use a clean cloth, wash it, and don't worry, it is natural – it is nothing to be scared of.'*

One of the BRAC health field staff responsible for supervising and monitoring teachers in the rural areas stated that some of the school teachers mentioned that in the past young girls would leave their menstrual cloths in inappropriate places. However, since learning about the need for hygienic practices during menstruation, they have kept their cloths in a proper manner, in a plastic packet or cloth wrapper, after washing and drying the material. Similarly, another BRAC staff member who has worked with the ARHE programme for several years mentioned that one of the most obvious impacts of the programme has been the adoption of hygienic practices by adolescent girls during menstruation.

While girls were especially interested in understanding menstruation, adolescent boys particularly wanted the ARHE to give them information related to sex, including AIDS, STDs, and family-planning methods. One of the boys explained the eagerness with which other adolescent boys approached him for answers about the female body and family-planning methods. He said: *'When my friends found out I was learning all of this in the school, they came and asked me a lot of questions, like "how does a girl get pregnant?" and "why do menses (periods) happen?" and "tell us about some family-planning methods"... I answered some of the questions. Not all, as I don't know many of the answers...'*

Family-planning methods were another popular topic with girls, which had until then been discussed mainly with friends, and in some cases with younger sisters-in-law or sisters. Except in a few rare cases, there was no discussion of family-planning methods between mothers and daughters. Adolescent girls said they were uncomfortable discussing these matters with their mothers and older female relatives, because communication patterns in rural Bangladesh are strongly influenced by gender and age. Family planning on the whole is a sensitive subject between older women and young unmarried girls in the 'traditional' rural culture (Mita and Simmons 1995).

Discussion about STDs and HIV/AIDS took place among the girls, but only one girl had talked about the issues with adults. Most of the girls were unclear about the causes and symptoms of the diseases, and thus sharing of knowledge with peers was confined to limited comments such as, 'If someone goes to a bad person (prostitute) they will get AIDS', or '[having] too many partners causes STDs'. Boys' knowledge of STDs and AIDS was also limited.

Adolescent boys were mainly interested in sharing what they had learnt in their ARHE classes with their friends and male cousins. One boy commented, 'At our age when the boys go to the bad place, they don't use condoms... I told my cousin that the illnesses [AIDS and STDs] spread if one does too much mixing. He became very quiet. I told him if he used condoms, as apa [teacher] had explained to us, he would prevent the illnesses from happening.' Another boy explained: 'What I found most important was family-planning methods – if we don't know this now, it can be damaging for us later. I told my friend – he studies in high school, and he does not know that if one does not use a condom when he goes to the bad place he can get AIDS.'

Wider dissemination of ARHE information

It is clear from the above that the newly acquired knowledge among adolescent boys and girls is also passed on to their peer networks in the villages. The adolescents who attend AHRE classes become an important source of basic knowledge about health for their unmarried and married peers, and for members of their families.

Some girls had also shared aspects of their new knowledge with their mothers. One mother remarked: 'My daughter and I talk about everything. She told me what to do if there is menstruation and how to keep myself clean. I am learning from her now.' Other mothers knew of their daughters' newly acquired knowledge about hygienic practices during menstruation, without having had an open discussion about it. One mother explained: 'I buy her soap, as she said she needs to wash her things with it. She asked me for the soap, so I got it for her but I don't say anything to her. What is there to say?

As long as she is learning all this, it is less worry for me, and she will know what to do.'

Girls' sharing of new knowledge of family-planning methods was confined to sisters-in-law[2] and close friends. 'I told my bhabi to use something – not to have too many children. I told her about the methods I had learned. She listened to me and asked me for more information, but I could only tell her what I knew. She said she would discuss it with my brother.' In one case, a girl discussed STDs with her older sister-in-law: 'I told her that if someone has an STD and has relations with his wife then she – the wife – can also get it, and the child can also be born with the illness.'

In all, the implementation of the ARHE programme within the schools, and the sharing of knowledge by adolescents via personal channels, have generated a new consciousness about reproductive health matters. The ARHE programme has to a certain degree legitimised 'making the unspoken spoken', in that the shame and silence surrounding girls' and boys' bodies has been broken, with the adolescents freely discussing 'taboo' subjects. Other studies of adolescent intervention programmes have also found that they result in adolescents 'break[ing] the culture and shame surrounding their bodies' (Mamdani 1998).

Love and romance

ARHE classes also seem to provide an opportunity for some adolescent girls and boys to share their feelings about *prem* (love) and 'romance'. This would have been considered unthinkable for previous generations in rural areas. In a culture where social interaction between a non-related adolescent male and female is disapproved of, and female virginity highly valued, the fact that adolescents – particularly females – are speaking about love shows a significant change in attitudes. In rural areas, if an adolescent girl is perceived to be behaving inappropriately – for example, not covering her body sufficiently modestly,[3] laughing and talking with boys or men, walking in a particular manner, being seen in 'public' spaces, and so on, she is subject to harassment, and the family faces dishonour as well. However, despite social pressure to conform, not all adolescents are following the norms.

Although some of the boys and girls said they wanted to make their own choices regarding their marriage partners, many admitted that their parents were the main decision-makers. Nevertheless, a number of adolescents said that they resorted to 'falling in love' secretly, in the hope of finding themselves a partner to marry, or in some cases, to elope with. However, usually these statements were accompanied by contradictory remarks such as 'good romance remains pure', or 'if two people like each other, then there is nothing wrong with the prem as long as it is not bad prem [sex is involved]'. Good love was defined as the boy and girl ultimately getting married to one another, and 'bad' or 'impure' love was defined as sex before marriage, or the boy and girl not marrying each other after having a relationship (even if it was 'pure').

Some adolescents said that boys initiate a relationship with girls through letters. Many of the boys' and girls' statements revealed emotions partly influenced by the romantic impressions made by movies, films, and television. In a culture where boys and girls have few opportunities to practise conversing in a romantic way, the popular films provide inspiration (Pelto 1999). A few of the boys and girls went beyond the letter stage and shared a kiss; another young couple went into town to take a picture of themselves; and another even went to the cinema together. Most couples resorted to meeting secretly after dark, in the fields or in empty schools, when family members were asleep.

Only a few adolescent girls and boys mentioned incidences of romances having happy endings. Situations such as these expose adolescent girls to particular risk, as they are far more vulnerable to coercive, unsafe, and unplanned sexual intimacies. Many of the female adolescents' narratives about the consequences of prem dwelt on betrayal, punishment from the village elders, jail, and unmarried girls getting pregnant. Some of the stories centred on revenge, where the girl was gang-raped, or acid was thrown to scar her face. Parents' stories mirrored that of the adolescents. However, their stories were tinged with anxiety and tension for their daughters: 'What to do if they (adolescents) run off and do bad work? How will we show our face in the village? We worry about our girls!'

Discussions of sexuality

The AHRE classes seem to have provided adolescent girls and women with a means of discussing sexuality. Young adolescent girls, and some of the teachers, were willing to speak out about their sexual desires, satisfaction, and needs with the researchers. This openness is particularly significant in a society where a woman or girl is seen as good and pure if she is sexually passive, and any overt expression of sexuality is considered shameful. One girl who spoke about sexual satisfaction said: 'My friend is very nice and he prays five times a day. He kissed me – I think that is normal ... Both men and women have equal rights in the sexual relationship.'

The language used by the teachers and adolescents implied that individuals are driven by some primal need, and are therefore not fully responsible for their own actions. Adolescent boys – and girls, too – mentioned that young people are unable to control their sexual urges, which usually leads to extra-marital activities. Some referred to 'too much desire/needs', and 'uncontrollable urges' brought on by hormones: 'Boys and girls get involved in sexual relations to meet their sexual needs.' This echoes another study in Bangladesh, in which several unmarried respondents blamed their sexual behaviour on 'urges', expressing a lack of personal responsibility for extra-marital sexual encounters (Caldwell and Pieris 1999).

A number of the boys in our study admitted to masturbating on a regular basis and did not appear perturbed, in contrast to another study which found that boys considered masturbation a sin (Hashima-e-Nasreen et al 1998). Masturbation was seen as something for *jonno mithano* (satisfying one's needs). Some boys mentioned spending time with their friends, watching pornographic films. *'We get together and watch all these naked people mixing with one another. We feel good, and we sit and masturbate to satisfy our desires.'* In Bangladesh, social attitudes towards sex and sexuality tend to be less rigid for boys than for girls. A mother spoke about her son's habit of watching blue films: *'They all get together and watch bf [blue films]... Sometimes I get angry and then they listen, but most of the time they do what they want.'* The other women participating in the discussion were smiling and whispering, and when the researcher asked the speaker if her daughter watched any blue films, all the women, including the mother, looked horrified. The mother stated: *'Girls don't watch such things. They would never do such things.'*

Adolescent boys appear to be aware that they have access to more sexual freedom and rights, compared with adolescent girls. While some boys felt that their behaviour was justified by the fact that they had *'more desires compared with adolescent girls'*, many commented that girls, although they may share similar urges and feelings, are unable to express themselves because of social pressures. Both the boys and girls stated that an adolescent girl, *'even if she is bursting to say or do something … will not do it'*.

Early marriage: adolescent girls asserting their rights

One topic in the AHRE curriculum is early marriage. In Bangladesh, adolescent marriage is exceptionally common. Parents and in-laws are the main decision-makers regarding young girls' entry into marriage and childbearing, and whether they will complete school (Caldwell and Caldwell 1998, cited in Gage 1998). In Nilphamari district, most girls are married off at 11–13, or even younger. In one of the schools in this district, we found that out of the 14 girls studying in the ARHE programme, six were already married, with two expecting their first children.

Despite widespread awareness of its detrimental effects on the health of girls and their babies, early marriage is still practised. According to mothers, the main reason for early marriage was the fear that their daughters would be 'spoilt', or raped, fall pregnant, or elope with a boy. Parents worry that while their daughters are studying in school they may be more at risk of sexual activity, as they have greater mobility and autonomy, and spend extended hours beyond the supervision of their families (Amin et al 1998). Adolescent girls tend to have limited mobility, particularly in poorer families, to safeguard their 'purity'. If the girl is known to have had pre-marital sex, the social status of the whole family is affected.

Many of the female adolescents who have participated in ARHE expressed reservations about early marriage, and are using their new knowledge about reproductive health to argue against early marriage. For example, during the research we found a girl imploring her mother: *'See – they are BRAC people, and they say early marriage is bad.'* Turning to us, she said: *'Look – why don't you explain to my mother that early marriage is bad for me?'* Later, when we were at her sister-in-law's home, she said to us: *'Tell her not to fix an early marriage for me. I should study more at school. Please don't get me married now.'*

The attitudes of some parents may be changing as they realise the advantages of more schooling for their daughters, as well as the dangers of early pregnancies. Some of the mothers admitted that they waited a little longer before marrying off their daughters, but confided that they faced harassment and derogatory comments from some elders in the community: *'Your girl has become big now, you should get her married... You are poor – what will she do with all this education?'*

Creating a network of peers

One feature of adolescence recognised by sociologists is the creation of a 'peer network' in which, through social inter-action, young people develop a sense of their own personal identity, as well as a group identity (Amin 1998, 196). The ARHE classes allowed interaction with classmates, with greater freedom from parental supervision. The changing values of the adolescents themselves have also led to changes in relations between female and male adolescents. Some of the girls' comments indicate that the classes have helped to dispel the awkwardness they felt previously, when interacting with the boys. In addition, they reported that a lot of the teasing had subsided. It seems that a 'comradeship' has developed in a few of the schools between some of the boys and girls.

Challenges for the ARHE programme

It is most important to remember that the ARHE is an innovative programme, which is functioning well in a strongly conservative environment, and still managing to provide adolescents with information on sexuality and reproductive health, no matter how basic. This should be viewed as a great achievement. However, there are some issues that need to be addressed in order to strengthen and improve the quality of the programme.

Teaching sensitive subjects to boys

In the final year of school, when ARHE classes are introduced, the health staff of BRAC assist and guide the teachers in teaching the curriculum. Due to time constraints and additional duties, their visits tend to be sporadic, and most of the responsibility is left to the school teacher. Some of the boys, initially taught by a member of BRAC's health staff, stated that after her visits decreased their teacher did not follow up and teach them the remaining curriculum.

The ARHE classes are given separately for boys and girls, because teachers and BRAC programme staff felt that it was culturally inappropriate to have boys and girls studying such sensitive subjects together. A teacher commented: *'When I first started teaching about puberty changes, they started laughing and giggling. The boys and girls started misbehaving ... After that, we decided that we would have separate classes for the boys and the girls.'*

One of the adverse effects of having separate classes is that some of the teachers were teaching the boys' classes infrequently. BRAC programme rules require that the classes are taught for an hour fortnightly in the schools. Interviews with some of the adolescent boys revealed that their classes were being held once a month, or less. When researchers raised this with two of the teachers, they admitted to having initial reservations about teaching such sensitive subjects, particularly to male adolescents. but had gradually become comfortable with teaching ARHE topics to adolescent girls. Most justified teaching girls on the basis of its being a duty, like that of an older sister. In contrast, they felt very uncomfortable about teaching the boys. One commented: *'I don't know about the other teachers of this programme, but I cannot teach the boys all these things. I feel ashamed.'* Some boys complained: *'Teacher doesn't teach explain to us properly about what we want to know, and we cannot ask her'.*

Gaps in knowledge of STDS, including HIV/AIDS

Most of the adolescents had only heard of 'the threat of AIDS', and saw it as a potential threat to the community, but not necessarily to themselves. While almost all the adolescents in the research were aware of the link between unprotected sexual intercourse and STDs and AIDS, and knew that condoms were an effective means of prevention, most also believed that 'immoral' people – prostitutes and men who behaved promiscuously – were the carriers of STDs and HIV.

There was a perception among all the adolescents that having multiple partners was risky. A common sentiment as expressed by one of the girls was: *'If someone goes to a bad person then AIDS happens... bad women who live without their husbands and have relations with other men – they have AIDS.'* Knowledge of how to prevent HIV/AIDS was incomplete and unclear. A common plea among students and teachers was: *'Please tell us in more detail so that we can learn how it happens and what happens. What are the symptoms of AIDS? How can we tell if someone has AIDS?'* Most of the adolescent boys and girls in the study appeared confused about the symptoms of HIV/AIDS and other STDs. Both adolescents and teachers said that if a person is affected with HIV/AIDS, she or he would show physical signs of illness.

The adolescents reported that the teachers preferred to focus mainly on menstruation, early marriage, and family-planning topics, and skimmed over the topic of STDs, including HIV/AIDS. One girl commented: *'Teachers don't explain to us clearly or openly about STDs and AIDS.'* This seems partly to relate to the shame and silence that has persisted around reproductive health matters but, more importantly, the teachers acknowledged that their own knowledge was weak, and blamed lack of detailed information in the ARHE curriculum.

Gaining wider community acceptance

In all the areas where the ARHE programme was set up, there were existing BRAC programmes, such as income-generating activities, non-formal schools, and micro-credit schemes. BRAC is a familiar organisation, and in some ways has become very much a part of the community. The teachers of the ARHE programme are selected from within the local community, and this, too, helps to gain acceptance for the programme. Also, most of the stakeholders in AHRE (students, teachers, parents, and community members) are involved in setting up the schools through which the ARHE is run: for example, by selecting the school site and deciding upon the school management committee.

Several other factors affect acceptance of ARHE in the community. Firstly, the mothers' knowledge[5] of the ARHE programme appears to be uneven. Many mothers knew about the ARHE programme and had detailed knowledge of the curriculum. At a discussion session, some of the mothers stated: *'They are learning so many important things, which we never had the chance to learn. It is important and very good that they are learning about family-planning methods. They can have small families in the future and be happy.'* However, some mothers are not aware of the content of all the classes. Boys tended to be too embarrassed to discuss sensitive subjects with their mothers. A majority of the adolescent girls preferred to discuss only the 'safer' topics with their mothers. A majority of the mothers were under the impression that their children were being taught *proiyojon* (necessary) life skills to prepare them for the future, but did not know in detail what these supposed life skills were. One adolescent explained: *'My parents don't really know in detail what we are being taught. We remain careful about what we say to them.'*

Power relations play a role in the acceptance of the programme. Most of the families from which ARHE participants come are very poor, and dependent on BRAC for educating their children. One boy explained the reasons why his mother did not protest: *'She is scared – what if they ask me to leave the school, if she complains? She doesn't want to anger the programme staff.'* Another reason could be that in a number of the areas the teachers of the school come from rich, influential families, some having direct links with authority figures in the village. Many poor people would feel uncomfortable questioning the 'authority' of a teacher who is not only educated but has a high social status.

Finally, with the increasing exposure of adolescents to outside influences, a large number of the mothers expressed worries that they were unable to control their adolescent boys and girls, and felt that 'life skills' and 'health education' were important for their children. Although some community members stated that providing information about reproductive health would encourage promiscuous behaviour, most have accepted the need for it. As one teacher and mother explained: *'This is the age when they make mistakes – so they need to know how to be careful...'*

Conclusion

Our research into the impact of the ARHE programme highlights the need for such education in rural areas. The programme provides information to young adolescent girls and boys in the programme, but also to other adolescents, and adults, who are not targeted by formal programme strategies. ARHE has mobilised the community, helping to break the silence and shame about 'sensitive' topics, and has thus affected relationships between adolescents and their parents, and among adolescents themselves. The diffusion of knowledge as a result of the ARHE is occurring in the context of a wider process affecting rural areas of Bangladesh, involving the media, books, exposure to urban and non-traditional ways of life, and schooling.

In future, additional research will be needed, with a greater focus on adolescents who participate in the programme and go on to marry. Will they be able to negotiate and decide on contraceptive methods together, and to what extent will their knowledge of reproductive health issues have a positive effect on their lives and the development of their communities?

Sabina Rashid is a research anthropologist working in the Research and Evaluation Division of BRAC (Bangladesh Rural Advancement Committee), Bangladesh, the largest non-government organisation in the world. Her postal address is A23 Century Estate, Bara Maghbazaar, Dhaka 1217, Bangladesh. Email: srashid@citechco.net

Notes

1 BRAC is one of the world's largest indigenous NGOs. Established in 1972, it has three main integrated but distinct programme areas: education, micro-credit, and health. The ARHE programme is under the umbrella of BRAC's health programme, the Health and Population Division (HPD).
2 The sisters-in-law are not much older than the adolescent girls themselves.
3 When discussing the issue of 'covering one's body', we are not referring to the veil but to the appropriate covering of one's arms, hands, legs, chest, and so on.
4 Interestingly, in most rural areas, the better-off families have televisions in their homes – and other families come over to watch programmes. Adolescent boys collect money and rent a television and video recorder from nearby video stores to watch pornographic films.

5 The fathers are usually busy and do not play a role in their children's education. It is mainly the mothers who attend the monthly school meetings, and they were always available at home when we went to interview.

References

Amin S, Diamond I, Naved R T, Newby M (1998), 'Transition to adulthood of female garment-factory workers in Bangladesh', in *Studies in Family Planning*, Vol. 29, No. 2

Caldwell B K and Pieris I (1999), 'Continued high-risk behaviour among Bangladeshi males', in J C Caldwell, P Caldwell et al, *Resistances to Behavioural Change to Reduce HIV/AIDS in Predominantly Heterosexual Epidemics in Third World Countries*, Health Transition Centre, Canberra

Gage, A J (1998), 'Decisionmaking regarding sexual activity and contraceptive use', in *Studies in Family Planning*, Vol. 29, No. 2

Hashima-e-Nasreen, Chowdhury M, Bhuiya A, Chowdhury S, Ahmed S M (1998), *Integrating Reproductive and Sexual Health into a Grassroot Development Programme*, BRAC-ICDDR, Bangladesh

Mamdani M (1999), 'Adolescent reproductive health: experience of community-based experiences', in Pachauri and Subramanian (eds), *Implementing A Reproductive Health Agenda in India: The Beginning*, Population Council, New Delhi

Mita R, and Simmons R. (1995), 'Diffusion of the culture of contraception: program effects on young women in rural Bangladesh', in *Studies in Family Planning*, Vol. 26, No 1

Nahar Q, Amin S, Sultan R, Nazrul H, Islam M, Kane T T et al (1999), *Strategies to Meet the Health Needs of Adolescents: A Review*, Operations Research Project, Health and Population Extension Division, Special Publications No.91, ICDDR, Bangladesh

Nahar Q, Huq N L, Reza, M, Ahmed, F (1999), Perceptions of Adolescents on Physical Changes During Puberty, ICDDR and Concerned Women for Family Development, Dhaka, Bangladesh (working paper, ICDDR)

Pelto P J (1999), 'Sexuality and sexual behaviour: the current discourse', in Pachauri and Subramanian (eds), *Implementing A Reproductive Health Agenda in India: The Beginning*, Population Council, New Delhi

Rashid S F and Michaud S (2000), 'Female adolescents and their sexuality: notions of honour, shame, purity and pollution during the floods', in *Disasters*, Vol. 24, No. 1,: pp.54–70

Acknowledgements

I would like to thank my colleagues Mahmuda Sarker, Nicci Simmonds, Dr Shamsher Khan, and Iftekar Khan for their assistance during project-designing and data-collection. For their useful comments and critical feedback I am grateful to my research coordinator, Fazlul Karim; my research colleague, Nusrat Chowdhury; and my husband, Safi Rahman Khan. I would also like to thank my field-research assistants for their hard work. I am grateful to the BRAC field-office staff for their assistance. Finally, my thanks to BRAC ARHE programme staff, adolescents, parents, and community members, who bore our endless questions with patience and humour.

Using life histories to explore change:

women's urban struggles in Cape Town, South Africa

Rachel Slater

This article examines the lives of four women who live in Cape Town, South Africa. Age and stage in the life cycle determined their ability to make a living in Cape Town, to survive shocking outbreaks of violence in the Crossroads squatter camp in 1983, and to avoid arrest under the 'pass laws' of the apartheid era. It shows how useful investigating people's life histories can be in developing understanding of the way in which their freedom to act is both constrained, and supported, by their context.

Anthropologists, sociologists, and historians have recorded and analysed people's life histories in their research for a long time (Denzin and Lincoln 1998). More recently, development researchers in both academic institutions and development organisations are using this technique increasingly frequently.

This article shows how life histories can be useful in analysing the impact of political and economic change on the lives of individuals and social groups. It draws on my own research in Cape Town, South Africa, which focuses on four black South African women and their experience of urbanisation. It starts by discussing life histories as a method for development research. From there, it moves on to outline the social, economic, and political context in which women migrated to Cape Town under apartheid.[1] Four case studies are used to highlight the shared, and individual, experiences of four women who arrived in Cape Town between 1949 and 1986, in defiance of the pass laws, which prohibited such migration.[2] The case studies show very clearly the structural constraints that have shaped these women's chances of making a livelihood. These constraints include not only the political, economic, and social limitations placed on black South Africans under apartheid, but also constraints related to gender and age. I argue that, regardless of the historical context, younger women were more successful in negotiating the daily struggle of urban township life than older ones who arrived in the city at the same time.

Using life histories in development research

Research into people's life histories has two particular strengths, which are especially important in the context of development.

First, life histories enable development researchers to understand how the impact of social or economic change differs according to the unique qualities of individual women or men. This is because they allow researchers to explore the relationship between individual people's ability to take action (their 'agency'), and the economic, social, and political structures that surround them. Researchers often choose to use alternative research methods – for example, structured interviews or surveys – to research the impact of change. However, these methods often lead to generalised results, which depict the experiences of 'ordinary people', suggesting that everyone experiences a particular event, trend, or policy in the same way (often irrespective of their gender). Using life histories 'humanises' development research, allowing us to challenge the tendencies to portray people as victims (Keegan 1988) or as happy peasants (Cross and Barker 1991).[3]

Life histories can be collected from women or men of similar or different ages, for different aims. For example, one researcher, examining older women's life strategies in South Africa, focuses on women born within a single decade (Bozzoli 1991). The research shows that women's migration and livelihood strategies have been constrained by their social, economic, and political context, but also shows that this context changes during the course of the women's lives. When they were young and single, the women in the research faced different opportunities and constraints in making a livelihood, compared with those facing them when they were older, with dependants. In contrast, the 14 women to whom I talked in my own research were drawn from a much wider range of ages. For example, Vuyelwa was 70 and had arrived in Cape Town in 1949, while Funeka, at 31, had been in Cape Town for just one decade. If women of different ages are interviewed, researchers are able to show the links between the different stages in the life courses of individual women, and the influence on those women of shifting economic contexts and historical changes as they occur at different stages of individual women's lives.

A second key strength of life histories in particular (and 'qualitative' research methods in general) is that they allow a much more open-ended interaction with people during an interviewing process. It seemed to me that talking to women about their lives in Cape Town was akin to freeing flood-waters that had been held back for years. These women were willing to tell their stories. A simple invitation to do so allowed the women themselves to define what was significant or crucial in shaping their experiences in the city. A structured questionnaire would not have yielded the same insights into the horrific violence that many women suffered at the hands of both African and white men, nor would women have felt free to tell their stories in any way they wished to.

Legal and economic constraints on women's movement to the city

This section briefly outlines the social, economic, and political context in which women migrated to Cape Town during the apartheid era.

A feature of urbanisation in South Africa has been the increasing presence of Africans in urban areas, despite legislative measures, commonly known as influx control, designed by the apartheid regime.[4] Influx control was intended to prevent Africans becoming anything more than temporary residents in cities.

In 1900, the African population of Cape Town was less than 10,000, most of whom were men employed at the harbour. The migrant labour system, already an entrenched policy of the government, was developed in the mines, but also used to regulate labour in Cape Town (Wilson 1972). In 1901, the outbreak of bubonic plague provided a 'dramatic and compelling opportunity for those who were promoting segregationist solutions to social problems', and Africans were removed from the city centre (Marks and Anderson 1987, 183). While the local authorities sought to remove Africans from Cape Town, processes of land alienation and forced removals under the 1913 Natives Land Act meant that more people sought work in the city. By 1920, manufacturing was established in Cape Town, and urban slums were developing at the city's periphery. The Natives (Urban Areas) Act of 1923 aimed to prevent Africans from entering and residing in cities, and it entrenched the notions of residential segregation and the principle that Africans were permitted into urban areas for labour purposes only (Davenport 1991). The 1923 Act applied to African men alone, as they formed the majority of migrants to Cape Town. Women and children remained in rural areas and relied on remittances from their husbands.

The Second World War and its aftermath saw rapid economic growth, matched by urban African population increase. A big demand for labour in Cape Town meant that influx control was implemented only half-heartedly (Nattrass 1981). However, a whole series of laws enacted in the 1950s later became the tool by which tens of thousands of people were moved out of Cape Town in the 1970s (Cole 1987). In 1950, the Population Registration Act required that all South Africans be classified according to racial origin. The predominance of the Coloured (mixed-race) population in Cape Town led the city and its hinterland to be classified as a Coloured Labour Preference Area (CPLA) in 1955 (Riley 1991). By protecting Coloured labour in the city, the government could further constrain African people from moving into the city.

Until 1952, women were not subjected to the laws that required African men to carry documents certifying their right to work and reside in urban areas. In 1952, the Natives (Abolition of Passes and Co-ordination of Documents) Act stipulated that all Africans over the age of 16 years were required to carry a reference book to be presented on demand to the police or pass inspectors.

The application of pass laws to women was to be central to their experiences of urbanisation, and would define their capacity to make a living for decades to follow. The intended impact of government policy on African women and family life was spelt out clearly in 1954 by the Cape Town City Council: 'The policy of this government is to reduce the number of African families in the Western Cape ... The labour needs of the peninsula are to be met by migratory labour ...Those who have the right to stay will be allowed to remain, the rest will go home' (quoted in Cole 1987, 7).

In the 1960s, shifts in the price of gold brought changing economic conditions in Cape Town. There was a stricter imposition of the Coloured Labour Preference Policy, and the South African government took stringent measures against illegal dwellers in Cape Town. But it was not until the 1970s that the economy took a sharp downward turn, and, for the first time since the 1920s, African population increase in the city outstripped economic growth (Preece 1994). The government launched a total onslaught on squatting in Cape Town. In the late 1970s and early 1980s, forced removals involved more people, and were enacted more brutally and destructively, than at any other time in the Cape. In the area called Crossroads, the government used divide-and-rule tactics to pitch one community of squatters against another. Eventually, the conflict boiled over when the *witdoeke*, an alliance of people identified by their white headscarves, attacked and burned down the shacks of other squatters in 1986 (Cole 1987)

In the townships, women became the primary targets of pass raids and harassment by the police. Women were the main targets of day-time raids on workplaces and of night-time and early-morning raids on hostels where they stayed illegally with their husbands. 'The Cape Peninsula is the only area in the country where more women than men are arrested under the pass laws ... It is clear that there is a special assault against women in the area in line with government policy of preventing African family life from taking further root in the Cape Peninsula' (West 1982, 467). This constant harassment had an enormous effect on women's daily struggles to work and to feed and clothe their families, as the following women's life stories will illustrate.

Stories of urban survival: four case studies

Vuyelwa

Vuyelwa was born in 1926 and grew up in Queenstown (a 'white' town between the so-called homelands of Transkei and Ciskei).[5] In 1949, as a young woman, Vuyelwa and her elder sister left to work in Cape Town, to escape their tyrannical, lazy father. Three years later, when the pass laws were first applied to women, Vuyelwa qualified automatically for a pass, and her right to work in Cape Town was endorsed. However, the fact that she was a legal worker did not affect the poor treatment that she experienced at the hands of her employers, which she remembers vividly:

'They (whites) were terrible that time. Before, when we were working for the white people, we had our dishes, our own dishes. We couldn't mix the dishes. It was because I was African and she was white. I couldn't wash them in the same bowl, I had to wash them outside.'

Vuyelwa worked and lived at the homes of white people for many years. She had three children, who were raised by her family at home. When her daughter, Sindiswa, came to visit, Vuyelwa moved to Gugulethu (an African township in Cape Town) to live

in the room of her 'homeboys' (other Africans from her home town). When Sindiswa became pregnant at the age of 20, they moved to a shack in Crossroads squatter settlement, where Vuyelwa found that she was often harassed by the police. Although she had a pass, she was still squatting illegally, and often had to evade arrest.

'... the white people didn't want us to stay there. We should run away. I remember the day I had just finished building my home. I got Sindiswa, and people said: "There are police!" I think it was about 8 o'clock in the evening. Well, I took my things, I took my bag and I ran away. I went to sleep for weeks there – we used to sleep in the bush. And then in the mornings I went to work and I washed at the train station and then I got a train and I got off there in Cape Town and went to the toilet. It was bad, very bad, and then I went to work. And I was with my ID, my pass. Even if you had the pass, they didn't want you staying there.'

In the 1970s, some of the former single-sex hostels in Langa (one of the first African townships in Cape Town, established in 1924) were transformed into homes for families. As a pass-holder, Vuyelwa applied for a house and, in 1979, was allocated one. At first, she did not like living in Langa: she found it too rough, and she knew few people. However, when violence escalated in Crossroads in the 1980s and the *witdoeke* forced thousands from their homes in KTC and Nyanga, she was thankful to have escaped.

Thokozile

Thokozile told me that she arrived in Cape Town in 1964, long after the imposition of the pass laws on women. Previously she had been working in a Transkei town, teaching the Xhosa language to Father Fisher, a priest. She came to Cape Town to be close to her mother, who had left the Transkei after being mistreated by her in-laws. Thokozile arrived in Cape Town without a pass, but, clutching a glowing reference from Father Fisher, secured employment in a hospital laundry. She called herself Virginia. The pass inspectors soon caught up with her.

'So I started work there – it was in January. In April, I saw two men standing in the laundry and they were asking for Virginia and I told them "I am Virginia", and they said "You are coming with us." I asked them why, and they said "You are not allowed to work here because you haven't got a pass."'

Thokozile found herself in a police cell. She was searched, her pockets were emptied, and she was told that she would be locked up that night and then taken to court in the morning.

'It was a terrible day that day. I will never forget it because it was hot outside, and everything was locked, and it was the first time I was locked up, and the window was so small. I was sweating. I didn't have anything to eat that day, for the whole day – I didn't eat until supper.'

The next day, Thokozile was sentenced to two months' imprisonment. After serving her sentence, she was escorted back to the Transkei by the wives of two African police officers. On arrival, she collected money that had been mailed to the post office from Cape Town by her boyfriend, bought a ticket, and caught the same train back to Cape Town along with her two escorts.

Thokozile was arrested on two more occasions. Each time, she was imprisoned and escorted back to the Transkei, where she bought a ticket straight back to Cape Town. At other times, she evaded arrest by sleeping in the bush, or by outwitting the inspectors who came to places of work and residence to check on passes. On one occasion, she saved herself from arrest by stripping naked and lying on a bed surrounded by women. When the pass inspectors burst through the door, they were confronted by the sight of Thokozile, seemingly in the late stages of labour, and they made a hasty retreat.

Thokozile eventually found stability in Cape Town, when Father Fisher found her a job as a cleaner at an adult education centre in Langa. She was taken to the administration office at Langa, to try to organise a pass.

'… in 1982, Sister Alfreda took me to Langa pass office. Mr Lawrence was working there, and he asked me "Where have you been all these years?" I told him "I have been playing hide and seek with the police!" And Mr Lawrence laughed, so he fixed my pass. I couldn't believe it. It was the first time I had the pass! From 1964 until 1982 I had been doing hide and seek with the inspectors.'

Nolindile

Nolindile could not tell me when she was born, but she had grown up in a remote part of the Transkei and was married there at the age of 18. For the first 20 years of their marriage, her husband Mackenzie worked at the mines near Johannesburg. He was dismissed when he contracted tuberculosis. For a while, farming supported the family, but the drought of the late 1970s turned Ngcobo into a dust-bowl. When his father's entire stock was wiped out by liver disease in the drought, Mackenzie went to seek work in Cape Town. Nolindile was reluctant for him to leave, because she feared he would find a new wife in the city.

'During the drought there was no water. Cattle, sheep, and goats were dying. Grass was dry. That is why he decided to come here. My heart was sore, because I didn't know whom he was going to stay with.'

For many years, Nolindile continued cultivating crops in Ngcobo, planting where there was a little moisture in the soil. Eventually, she became ill and could not be cured by the local traditional doctor. Mackenzie sent money to finance a journey to Cape Town. In Cape Town, Nolindile was diagnosed at a local hospital with a kidney infection; but her illness was to be the least of her worries. She found Mackenzie squatting in Crossroads, and was immediately confronted with the escalating violence there.

'When I came here in 1986, there was a big fight in Crossroads. Then I thought to myself, why should I come here, because I didn't even know about this fight?'

Nolindile was bewildered by the town life that she encountered in Crossroads. Her only role in the city appeared to be to do the washing, since she did not have to go to the fields or collect wood and water. She says she has nothing else to do each day:

'Life changed now, because up country I used to wake up very early, and now I wake up any time I like, not very early. I wake up, make myself breakfast, do the washing, and then there is nothing else I can do. Up country I was working the whole day.'

In spite of her best efforts to find employment in Cape Town, Nolindile has never worked in the city. She has never been to school, has no experience of wage labour, speaks no language except Xhosa, and still has many children to look after. In 1995, she also was diagnosed with tuberculosis, the illness that had forced Mackenzie out of work in the late 1960s. The daily treatment that she endured for a year cured her of tuberculosis, but she remains sickly to this day and has all but abandoned hope of finding employment.

Funeka

Funeka, a 31-year-old living on a site-and-service stand,[6] is the focus of my fourth case history. For Funeka, living in Cape Town has been a succession of moves, each time as a refugee fleeing waves of intense conflict and violence. She came to the city from rural Transkei in 1986, after an unsuccessful marriage. First, she stayed just outside Cape Town, where her stepfather worked, and lived in the hostels owned by fruit companies, who relied on cheap labour to harvest and process deciduous fruits. She stayed there for some time, pretending to be 'Coloured', so she could work packing apples. The fruit factories were within the Coloured Labour Preference Area, so it was difficult to find work as an African. At night, she often had to flee the hostels to avoid the pass inspectors. Eventually it became too difficult to avoid arrest there, and she moved to Crossroads in 1986. She arrived in the midst of the Crossroads conflict, and stayed three years.

'In Crossroads, I started a business. I was selling meat and beers. We stayed nice and quiet in Crossroads. Oh! Then the violence erupted, our houses were burnt down. We stayed in Nyanga centre for four months. We had lost everything. We were moved to Site C, and then again in Site C there was violence. Then we ran to Greenpoint, then from Greenpoint to Macassar here.'

In Greenpoint, Funeka lived with her brother, a taxi-driver, until he was killed in a 'taxi war' – a conflict between rival operators of public mini-buses. One day, a group of men burst into the shack where Funeka lived with her brother, and pulled him outside. They then set upon him with knives, poured paraffin over him and set him alight. He was burnt alive. Fearing for her own safety, Funeka ran away, but returned a month later to try to collect together some of her belongings.

She successfully registered for a new site-and-service stand in Macassar, fleeing from violence for the third time in less than ten years.

At the time I met her, in 1996, Funeka was living in Macassar, Khayelitsha, an area of Cape Town established in 1983. She lived with her son Vusumzi and her brother. Peter, Vusumzi's father, also lived with them, but often disappeared for days on end. He rarely gave Funeka money for food; she relied heavily on income made from sewing, and money contributed by her brother. Funeka was not in love with Peter; with no illusions about her relationship with him, she was honest about its limited benefits.

'The main reason why (I wanted to have a boyfriend): I was alone. I built this house. I had no boyfriend. Now, there was a girl staying alone, and her house was burnt down, and no-one saved this girl. If there was a man, he should have saved her, and there is this breaking-in of skollies (vandals) at night. I was also afraid of that. Well, I decided to have somebody to stay with.'

After years of forced removals, evading the pass laws and being shunted from pillar to post to escape appalling violence, it is not surprising that Funeka views Khayelitsha as a city of broken people. However, she is finally finding some peace in Macassar. Perhaps because she is the youngest of the women whose life stories I collected, her feet seem to be firmly rooted in town. In spite of the endemic violence, unrest, and poverty that characterise life in Khayelitsha, I felt that Funeka somehow maintained the energy to keep going, whatever life threw at her.

Gender, age, and life-stage: shaping women's lives

When I looked in detail at these four women's experience of apartheid policies in an urban setting, it became clear that other factors beyond the immediate social, economic, and political context have shaped their lives. These are gender, age, and the stage of life that women had reached when factors in the external context affected them.

Comparing the four stories, it is clear that certain aspects of South Africa's influx controls affected all the women *as women*. There was a distinct gender dimension to urban apartheid. Women were the targets of most pass raids in the townships, hostels, and squatter camps, and occupied a much more precarious position in the city than men. The policy of influx control approved the presence of limited numbers of African men in cities as temporary labour, and the authorities had built single-sex hostels to accommodate them. The fact that African women were not welcome was reflected in the limited family housing that existed in the two townships of Gugulethu and Nyanga. This housing was very overcrowded. During the Crossroads conflict, the South African government set women against men, in order to divide communities. It actively undermined the women's group that sought to find a solution to the conflict, and supported the *witdoeke* as they attacked other squatters (Cole 1987). Women of all ages were very vulnerable to attack by the *witdoeke*, and to rape and sexual assault.

Women's ages, and the stages they had reached in their life cycles, were determining facts in their experience of arrival and survival in Cape Town. Vuyelwa and Funeka were both very young when they arrived, and both seemed to have adapted relatively easily to town life. Vuyelwa's path was made easier because she automatically qualified for a pass on arrival in 1949, but both she and Funeka, who arrived in 1986, were better equipped to cope with nights in the bush and evade pass inspectors, particularly because neither had small children to look after. Both were seeking social and financial independence from their families, and may well have fared better for feeling much less loyalty and responsibility towards their families in the Transkei than older women.

In contrast, women arriving at an older age had usually come to Cape Town at a moment of crisis, fleeing dire economic conditions in the Transkei. They had stronger family ties and a sense of responsibility for children and other dependants. Consequently their sense of the need to support people back in the Transkei was much stronger. Of the four women above, Nolindile had struggled through illness and years of drought at home before moving to Cape Town with her children, leaving other family members behind. Thokozile abandoned her job in the Transkei after several months of loneliness, following family problems and her mother's departure.

Age and stage in the life cycle were important also in the sense that the length of time that women spent in Cape Town influenced their capacity to seize opportunities that came their way, or find their way around constraints affecting residence and employment. As described earlier, one common effect of apartheid policies in Cape Town was the shortage of housing for Africans. However, while all the women had problems in establishing secure, stable homes, these difficulties were compounded for those with fewer years' experience in Cape Town. When I met them, Thokozile (who arrived in 1964) and Vuyelwa (who arrived in 1949) occupied brick houses with full services, while Nolindile and Funeka, who both arrived in 1986, lived on site-and-service stands, at risk from annual flooding in the winter months. The women's ability to get access to housing was dependent on a series of prerequisites, such as whether they had children, possessed passes, or could call on people from the same area of the Transkei who now lived in Cape Town. Married couples – with or without children – who possessed passes could apply for family housing in Gugulethu. Younger, unmarried women without children could often find accommodation with homeboys, but the homeboys were frequently reluctant to house older women or women with children, who were viewed as a greater burden.

Conclusion

Each of the women's stories that are presented here has painted a different picture of the experience of migration to Cape Town and survival in urban areas under apartheid. The technique of analysing women's life stories shows that there are common aspects in their experience, some of which are related to their gender, age, and life stage; in addition, there are aspects that are unique to particular women. Funeka and Thokozile come across as having both the strength of character and the adaptability to respond to changing opportunities and constraints on life in Cape Town, while Nolindile did not seem to adapt to town life at all. Thus, it is difficult – if not impossible – for a researcher to understand the impact of particular policies or development interventions by untangling common experiences from those that are unique. Urban apartheid and influx control governed the working and social lives of all the women, but not necessarily in the same manner, at the same time, or to the same extent. It is only possible to understand women's experiences of urbanisation by analysing the way in which factors particular to individuals, such as age and stage in the lifecycle, cross-cut the structural context that shapes women's lives.

So what are the implications of this for policy-makers and planners in development? It seems to me that the use of life histories in development research enables us to examine the impacts of policies on different kinds of people, rather than homogenising people's experiences of poverty and the ways in which a policy affects them. Furthermore, life histories offer a good opportunity to inject humanity into our analyses of social and economic change.

Rachel Slater is Research Officer at the Institute for Development Policy and Management, University of Manchester, Crawford House, Precinct Centre, Oxford Road, Manchester, M13 9GH, UK E-mail: rachel.slater@man.ac.uk

Notes

1 Apartheid was the policy of separate development for people of different racial groups (black, white, 'Coloured' and Indian) in place in South Africa from 1948 until the first fully democratic elections in 1994.

2 The 'pass laws' were laws enacted and amended from 1923 onwards that governed the residence and movement of blacks in South Africa. The main objective of the laws was to prevent the entrance of blacks into South Africa's urban areas, except where and when their labour power was required.

3 'Victims' are people viewed as having no agency and whose lives are determined by the structures that surround them. The idea of 'happy peasants' suggests people who, despite their impoverished state, are unaware of the hardships that they endure and the social, political, and economic inequalities that straddle all parts of the globe.

4 In the South African context, the term 'African' is used historically to denote the black population, since the South African government renamed Africans as 'blacks', 'natives' and 'bantu' at various times. It is not meant to suggest that white or Coloured South Africans are not African.

5 The 'homelands' were areas reserved for African settlement under apartheid in which Africans of particular tribal groups were expected to subsist through agriculture. These areas were an important source of surplus labour for the mines and South Africa's urban areas.

6 A plot of land with water and electricity supplies laid on.

References

Bozzoli, B (1991), *Women of Phokeng: Consciousness, Life Strategy and Migrancy in South Africa, 1900–1983*, Ravan Press, South Africa

Cole, J (1987), *Crossroads: The Politics of Reform and Repression, 1976–1986*, Ravan Press, South Africa

Davenport, T R H (1991), *South Africa: A Modern History*, Macmillan, UK

Keegan, T (1988) *Facing the Storm: Portraits of Black Lives in Rural South Africa*, David Philip Publishers, South Africa

Marks, S and Anderson, N (1987), 'Issues in the political economy of health in South Africa', *Journal of Southern Africa Studies*, Vol. 13, No.2, pp.175–86

Preece, H (1994), 'The economics of apartheid' in Harker, J, *The Legacy of Apartheid*, Guardian Newspapers, UK

Nattrass, J (1981), *The South African Economy: Its Growth and Change*, Oxford University Press, UK and South Africa

Riley, E (1991), *Major Political Events in South Africa, 1948–1990*, Oxford University Press, Facts on File

Slater, R (1998), 'Putting Down Roots: African Women's Lives and Livelihoods in the Townships of Cape Town, South Africa', PhD Thesis, Institute for Development Policy and Management, University of Manchester

West, M (1982), 'From pass courts to deportation: changing patterns of influx control in Cape Town', *African Affairs*, No. 81, pp.463–77

Wilson, F (1972), *Migrant Labour in South Africa, Johannesburg*, South African Council of Churches

Intact or in tatters?

Family care of older women and men in urban Mexico

Ann Varley and Maribel Blasco

This article asks how family relationships affect the living conditions of low-income elderly people in urban Mexico. There is little State provision of accommodation for the elderly, forcing older people to rely on their families for care. Yet many poorer families cannot afford to provide care, and some are unwilling to do so. In addition, families treat elderly men and women differently, with significant consequences for women's and men's housing conditions and wellbeing in later life.

The material that we analyse comes from a three-year research project on gender and housing in Guadalajara, Mexico's second-largest city.[1] The research has a variety of aims. One of them is to identify new directions for gender-sensitive policy formulation. We also plan to produce a small publication for grassroots and non-government organisations working from a gender perspective, looking at how housing issues can be incorporated into the empowerment process. In Guadalajara, our work focused on four low-income neighbourhoods that we considered offered all the main housing options open to the low-income population. The first was a recent self-help settlement on the edge of the city; the second was a similar settlement dating from the 1950s; the third, a government-housing project of apartment blocks; and the fourth, an inner-city area with a high proportion of rental housing. In each area, we organised discussion groups with residents: one of women, one of men. Each group met on six occasions, discussing a variety of topics. In addition to the eight discussion groups and individual follow-up interviews, we conducted two questionnaire surveys in each area, concerning individual housing histories and the broader response to issues discussed in the groups. Finally, we undertook interviews in several *asilos* (homes for the elderly). The names of people quoted have been changed.

The caring family as safety-net for the elderly

The proportion of the population aged over 60 is rising in developing countries. The question of who will care for these growing numbers of elderly has, until recently, been neglected (Tout 1989). It is often assumed that the family will automatically take on this responsibility, yet little is known about the reliability of this safety net in practice (de Vos 1990).

In Mexico, strong family ties are often thought to be a distinguishing feature of the national soul, and the family is popularly seen as an unfailing source of support to its members. The possibility that families might refuse to care for elderly relatives is seemingly too remote to be worth considering (see, for example, Contreras de

Lehr 1992). This myth of the ideal family is a persistent one, but many elderly people cannot, in fact, rely on their families for housing and support. Some of those who are housed by relatives are neglected or abused: the family is not always an ideal solution. Yet idealisation of the caring family provides hard-pressed governments with a pretext for them to pass the buck to relatives, expecting them to care for the elderly with minimal support from health or welfare services.

The mistaken belief that the family will automatically support its members is reflected in the lack of institutional provision for the elderly. In Guadalajara, demand for *asilos* has increased dramatically over the last decade or so, far outstripping supply. This is particularly problematic for low-income elderly people. Few *asilos* are free, and for the very poor, who usually do not receive pensions, even a small charge is prohibitive. It is estimated that of tomorrow's elderly population (those currently 45–65 years old), only 42 per cent will be covered by some form of social security provision (Montes de Oca, 1999). The institution that caters for the most vulnerable sectors of the elderly population is the DIF (*Desarrollo Integral de la Familia* – 'Integral Family Development'). However, the DIF attends to only a few hundred elderly people in its *asilos* in each of the major cities.

Another unfortunate consequence of the ideology of the responsible family is the belief that if you are not cared for by your children, you must have done something in earlier life to merit the otherwise inexplicable treatment of being left to fend for yourself. When we asked the personnel of *asilos* why elderly people live in these homes, they sometimes suggested that the residents had somehow deserved this fate. The director of a home for abandoned elderly men and women told us: *'It's always said that what you sow is what you'll reap'* (interview, Guadalajara, May 1998).

In the following discussion, we explore some of the housing options available to the elderly, and some of the things that can render older women and men vulnerable.

Living alone or with family: differences between women and men

In 1990, nearly two-thirds of older people living alone in Mexico were women. Nearly one in ten women of 60 years or more was living alone.[2] Women's greater longevity means that there are more older women than older men, but those living alone outnumber men even more. There were 112 women for every 100 men of 60 years or more, but 170 (and as many as 224 in the largest urban areas) for every 100 men living alone.

The existence of so many elderly women living alone in Mexico is at odds with cultural beliefs portraying mothers as the archetypal recipients of family charity. Mothers are supposed to be objects of near-veneration for their children. This has been used to help to explain census data revealing that elderly women enjoy better physical housing conditions than their male counterparts. The family is thought to be 'more willing to provide help or financial support to their mother or female relatives than to their father or male relatives' (Llera Lomelí 1996, 166).

Since family care for elderly women is taken for granted, those who, for whatever reason, live alone are particularly vulnerable to being judged as 'reaping what they have sown'. If Mexican children do not support their mother in her old age, she 'must' have been a bad mother. So, in addition to their precarious living conditions, older women may have to face being blamed for being 'rejected' by their family. Those who have never married – because of their sexual preferences, for example – are also vulnerable to this type of moralising, since they may be seen as having failed in the task of developing 'normal' bonds of affection with others that will sustain them in later life. The proportion of never-married women in *asilos* is far greater than any other category, suggesting that childless women are the most vulnerable group among elderly women.

Why do women live alone more frequently than men? It is well known that they live longer. In Mexico, women generally marry men a few years older than them, and they are less likely than men to re-marry if they are divorced or widowed. Older women are therefore less likely than men to have a surviving spouse. In 1990, 76 per cent of men of 65 years or over were married or living with a partner, compared with only 44 per cent of older women (López and Izazola 1994).

Thus, older women are more likely to live alone, partly because of their longer life expectancy, which increases their chances of finishing their lives without a partner. This observation leaves unanswered, however, the question of why these women are not living with relatives.

Our work in Guadalajara suggests that elderly women may increasingly be forced to fend for themselves as a result of changes in family relations and female employment patterns. In Mexico, as elsewhere, it is younger women who have typically cared for elderly relatives (Lloyd-Sherlock 1997). Yet women's role as carers can no longer be taken for granted, due to their increased participation in the labour market. This, coupled with greater access to schooling, has led to changes in younger women's attitudes, so that they no longer unquestioningly submit to their husbands' wishes (LeVine with Sunderland Correa 1993).

Many younger women now object vociferously to living with their in-laws. There is a long history of poor relations between mother-in-law and daughter-in-law, creating lasting bitterness, as traditionally the older woman has taken it on herself to teach the younger one to 'know her place'. As Mexico has changed from a rural to an urban society, the country has seen a growing rebellion against that tradition. As one younger woman told us: *'Women were more submissive in the past – if they were taken to live with their husband's parents, they stayed put and didn't protest. Nowadays they rebel, so when he says "We're going to live with my mother", they reply, "No way! Your mother doesn't like me – go and find me a place where we can be on our own" ... I think it's because women work now, and we feel we have more right to have our say'* (group discussion, older self-help settlement, Guadalajara, November 1997).

Older women can therefore no longer rely on living with their married sons. Neither can they count on living with their married daughters. According to one social worker whom we interviewed in a State-supported home for elderly people, women who do not have jobs find it difficult to persuade their husbands to house their mothers (interview, Guadalajara, May 1998).

There is a flaw in some discussions of older people living in extended households, which assumes that the elderly have moved in with their children. This reflects a widespread tendency to view older people as passive and dependent, and ignores the important question of whose house it is. There is a considerable social and psychological difference between having a son-in-law or daughter-in-law move in with you, and moving in with a married child and his or her family. We therefore sought to see which of these situations was more common in the areas where we were working. Our questionnaire survey yielded individual information on only a small group of older people: 131 people of 60 years or over. It is interesting, however, because we distinguished between those with and without a partner, and between those who were living in a house they owned or had rented and those who were living in someone else's house.

We found, as expected, that more men (82 per cent) than women (50 per cent) still had partners, while more women (10 per cent) than men (3 per cent) lived alone. But while almost one-quarter of women without a partner (11 per cent of all the women) were living with a son's or daughter's family, no men were doing so. Three-fifths of the men were still living in their own homes with their wives or wives and children. In all, 17 per cent of women were living in a relative's house, but only 5 per cent of men. In short, older men are more likely to be cared for by their spouses in their own homes, whereas women are more likely than men to live alone or be 'taken in' by adult children.

Not being a burden, or getting some peace: older women on their own

Significantly, although living alone is generally negatively portrayed, many women whom we interviewed said that this would be their preferred housing option when elderly. Living alone clearly has certain practical disadvantages, such as not having any one around if you are suddenly taken ill. Even having family nearby, as many people do, is not necessarily going to solve that problem. Women in the oldest age groups are more likely to be infirm and in need of medical attention, and most at risk on their own. Their alternatives are also more limited, as the social worker in a State-supported home mentioned earlier told us: many *asilos* will not admit people who are incapacitated – *imposibilitadas* – or ill (interview, Guadalajara, May 1998).

In addition, people can clearly suffer problems of loneliness and low self-esteem resulting from internalisation of the notion that 'what you sow, you reap'.

In spite of these disadvantages, over two-thirds of the women aged 60 or more with whom we spoke in Guadalajara said that they would prefer to carry on living in their own homes as they grew older. Although most wanted to be with their children or husbands, just over one in ten specified 'alone'.[3] When asked why they should want to live alone, women (of all ages) often said they wouldn't want to 'make a nuisance' of themselves. A few explicitly mentioned not wanting to have problems with their daughters-in-law, or to cause trouble between their daughters and sons-in-law. Some (although fewer of the older women) said they'd rather be in a home, *'so my children don't get tired of me, and so as not to be a burden'* (questionnaire survey, Guadalajara, April 1998).

It is tempting to see these responses as expressing the traditional feminine ideal of self-denial (*abnegación*). They should not, however, always be taken at face value, as they may conceal women's own fears and concerns – particularly about having to look after the grandchildren. Some women were happy to say straight out that they didn't want this: *'on my own, so no-one can cause me any trouble'*, or *'on my own, so I don't have to be battling, either with my daughters-in-law or with my grandchildren'*. They had worked hard enough bringing up their own children in poverty, and felt they deserved a break. For others, however, 'not wanting to be a burden' expressed, indirectly, a complaint about being expected to look after their grandchildren or do housework for their children's families (Varley and Blasco, 1999).

'Fathers are two a penny': older men's problems

Older men are far less likely to live alone or be dependent on relatives for care than women. During their lives they have had greater access to education, formal-sector employment, pensions, and health care.

More men than women work, mirroring employment patterns in earlier life. As we have seen, older men are more likely to have surviving spouses than women. Consequently, they are less likely to live alone during the final years of their lives. They are less frequently dependent on relatives and are usually financially better off (Llera Lomelí 1996, INEGI 1993).

Our research nonetheless revealed some unexpected problems that elderly men can face. As with women, many of these problems derive from constraints and cultural norms operating at earlier stages in their lives. We found that those men who do become dependent in old age can experience more extreme destitution than women, for several reasons.

According to both older and younger men in our study, Mexican men's most significant role is still that of breadwinner. Men who cannot live up to this ideal risk losing their family's respect, and their own self-esteem. Being a good father, and therefore a good man, depends on being a good provider. Other contributions that a father may make, such as providing care and nurturing, may not be highly valued. Widespread poverty means, however, that many men are unable to fulfil their breadwinner role adequately. In old age, a man who has barely been able to scrape a living has few bargaining counters, since respect for fathers is often based on largely material considerations. He cannot always offer his children a house or other inheritance, in exchange for their caring for him.

Moreover, the need to earn a living in harsh circumstances means that most low-income men spend little time with their families. Ironically, the pressure to provide prevents men from developing good relationships with their children. Older men may find that, having failed to invest emotionally in their families during their working lives, they are rejected when they need support. Whereas being a mother is

success in itself, being a father is not enough on its own. As one 68-year-old grandmother put it in one of the group discussions: *'Fathers are two a penny, but mothers don't grow on trees.'*

Divorced and separated fathers, and men who have children with different women or abandon young families, are all particularly at risk of rejection by their children when they become elderly. As responsibility for child-care after a separation almost always falls to the woman, men's links with their children can be very fragile, or non-existent. Should a man abandon his family or behave abusively towards them, he cannot count on receiving support in later life.

Furthermore, relatives may be less willing to take in elderly men, since they are perceived as incapable of carrying out child-care and housework and thus 'paying' for their keep. Men may also find it more difficult to fit into another household. When a man is taken into a married female relative's household, her husband may resent the attention she gives to the older man. Men are also regarded as less morally 'trustworthy', and their sexual behaviour as questionable, regardless of their age, as men from the older self-help settlement said:

Jaime (aged 67): *No one's going to trust a man, no matter how old he is. He won't be trusted in anyone's home.*

Jesús: *You never know what mañas* [habits; with strong sexual overtones] *he might have.*

Jaime: *But with a woman it's different. They adapt better. People say: 'You can stay here if you haven't got anywhere to go.' Anyone will be willing to take them in. Any family. But with a man – no-one's going to take him in anywhere, and less still if he's a dirty old devil* [mañoso].

If men are indeed less capable of looking after themselves and the home, they will also find it more difficult to cope with living alone in old age. In Mexico, and other countries, older men are documented as receiving less help from children, and having less contact with other kin than elderly women (Llera Lomelí 1996, Barer 1994). They also tend to be more readily isolated from their families and social networks by bereavement, owing to weaker relationships in earlier life. As one respondent put it: *'It's more difficult for an elderly man to live alone, because people visit women a lot more.'* All these factors can threaten men's well-being in old age.

Living with family: a haven for the elderly?

Living with family is usually thought to be a better option for older people. However, we should not assume that this guarantees their well-being. In Mexico, we heard of cases where elderly people had been physically or emotionally abused at the hands of their relatives.

Although we have suggested that owning a home gives older people a 'bargaining counter' to exchange for care from relatives, it can make them more vulnerable to abuse. When we asked discussion-group members whether or not older people should put their children's name on property documents, the men in the younger self-help settlement immediately responded 'no!' – because, said one, *'they'll chuck you out'*. Both women and men cited examples of children cheating or trying to cheat their parents of their property, and the staff of government agencies legalising land tenure in self-help settlements told us of others. Most low-income people who own a housing plot in urban Mexico acquire the land illegally. Too often, people registering their property in a son's or daughter's name have ended up 'out on the street'.

Of course, living with children is not always such a gloomy experience. It can be an invaluable housing option, particularly

for the very elderly. Many children have genuine affection for their parents, and feel morally obliged to help them. A woman in the older self-help settlement identified a sense of obligation towards her parents as a specifically female responsibility, and even a right: *'We women take care of our parents when they get old, because they're our parents, it's our right and our duty to take care of them.'*

Others expressed the responsibility to look after their parents in terms of a 'do-as-you-would-be-done-by' logic: *'The way you treated that person, that's the way they're going to treat you.'* This moral accounting sometimes takes the form of an explicitly Catholic morality: *'building up your stock of virtue in heaven'*, as one 68-year-old grandparent put it.

Some interviewees expressed appreciation of elderly people's 'folk knowledge': stories from the past, recipes, herbal remedies, and other lore that might otherwise be lost. This intangible contribution to family life was one of the main reasons that people gave for wanting to care for older relatives.

The flow of benefits in the relationship is not, then, always unidirectional, with elderly parents on the receiving end. Children may remain with their parents because they cannot afford independent accommodation. Some stay in the hope that they will be left the house when their parents die. There has been a tradition of the youngest son remaining at home, caring for his parents and subsequently inheriting the property. Although this is normally described as a rural tradition, women with whom we talked in the inner city agreed that it was usual to leave property to either the youngest child or a daughter or son who had cared for their parents.

Grandparents, especially grandmothers, often fulfil important functions within their children's household. They frequently help out with household chores or care for grandchildren to enable another family member to go out to work. While these activities may be tiring for the elderly person, they can also help them to feel that they are 'paying their way'. Accounts of mutually beneficial relationships between parents and children sharing accommodation should not, however, be taken at face value. The idea of symbiosis, though appealing, should be treated with some scepticism. At a workshop at which we discussed these issues, one participant who had worked on social provision for older people in Mexico City commented that listening carefully to women talking about their role within a relative's home may reveal insecurity and even fear behind the rhetoric of mutual support. The gratitude they express towards their relatives could be better described as a *'gratitud-esclavitud'* (slavery-gratitude). Some women who were initially enthusiastic about support groups that he had organised for them did not, in practice, turn up. He later learned that they were afraid to leave their daughters' homes or neglect their domestic work (International Research and Policy Workshop on Reducing Vulnerability Among Families in the Mexico and US Border Region, Desarrollo Integral de la Familia (DIF) Nacional and University of Texas, Tijuana, March 1999).

As the authors of a study of women's lives in Cuernavaca have written, 'poorer women were having to make themselves as useful as possible to adult children, thereby building up credit for the time when their health failed and they could no longer "earn their keep"' (LeVine with Sunderland Correa 1993, 193).

The *asilo*: attractive option or prison sentence?

We have noted that the amount of accommodation on offer in *asilos* is very limited; but how do people in Guadalajara respond to the idea of spending their later years in a home? We found that men and women reacted very differently to the prospect. Many women said they would like to live in a home: retaining their independence, resting, and receiving the care they need. Men, on the other hand, flatly rejected the *asilo* for being 'like a prison', where they would be badly treated.

Men's objection to institutional accommodation reflects their feelings about the (family) home. Many find it difficult to relate to the home, because they spend so little time there during their working lives, and because culturally the home is the woman's sphere. 'Men are for the street and women for the home', as a Mexican saying puts it. Many men we spoke to appeared to feel far more 'at home' at work: when we asked older men to tell us about the houses they had lived in over the course of their life, they often turned the conversation around to their work, not housing, history.

The things that make it hard for elderly men to adapt to the home also make it difficult for them to adapt to *asilo* life. Homes for the elderly are generally run by women, often nuns. Men can feel out of place in an environment where women are in control, and *asilo* rules are anathema to them, because they have been used to coming and going as they please. *'Men want to be free, they want to go wherever they like,'* one *asilo* director told us: *'They're not used to being at home all the time, they always want to be free, right?'* (interview, Guadalajara, May 1998). Institutional life drives home to men the fact that that they are now dependent, and they can experience this as an affront to their dignity. As the director of an *asilo* for men told us, *'Here they have to obey the rules and schedule. That's very hard for them and some of them never get used to it'* (interview, Guadalajara, May 1998).

Reluctance to face life in an institution may lead some men to end up on the streets. In a study of vagrants in Mexico City, almost four out of five were found to be men, with an average age of 53 (Montes de Oca 1999). Older men may also be less welcome in mixed *asilos* than women. According to staff, they are more troublesome: more often violent and even sexually abusive. The director of one home for older women in Guadalajara told us: *'No one wants to look after men, even in their own homes. Women are loved more than men. Men are more difficult in every respect'* (interview, Guadalajara, May 1998).

Institutional accommodation is not, then, always a viable solution for older men. Its combination of home-like and institutional characteristics makes it unpopular with them, as they are unaccustomed to having their freedom curtailed. Women's greater willingness to contemplate life in an *asilo* may express both the desire to 'retire' from a life of domestic labour, and the knowledge that women generally survive their husbands, and few can rely on being cared for by their spouses. Perhaps seeing other women widowed leads women to think about their own options for the future more seriously than men.

Conclusion

In his book *Ageing in Developing Countries*, Ken Tout remarks on his impression that the saddest individual experience tends to be that of the widowed aged man, particularly where incompetence in domestic matters aggravates his abandonment. But, *en masse*, it is elderly women who are more likely to suffer problems (Tout 1989, 289).

Our research in Guadalajara supports this conclusion. While it is widowers abandoned by relatives whose plight may be most acute, it is older women living alone who represent the greater challenge for social policy: there are more of them. We have seen that elderly women are more likely than men to live with, or be taken in by, married sons or daughters and their

families. It is ironic, however, that the very skills that enable older women to 'fit in' also make it easier for hard-pressed relatives to feel that they will be all right on their own.

Researchers often warn against the dangers of translating policy prescriptions from one cultural context to another. It is tempting to interpret the strong cultural emphasis on family solidarity in Mexico as meaning that older people would be happiest living with their relatives. We have tried to show that this is not necessarily the case, and that we should not always take what people say on this matter at face value. We are not suggesting that we know better than older Mexican women and men what is in their best interests. To do so would be both unacceptably arrogant and extremely foolish. What we are saying is that it is important to listen very carefully to exactly what people are saying. When your feelings are at odds with cultural norms – for example, about mothers putting their family first – you may half-hide them behind a façade that is more culturally acceptable. 'Not wishing to be a burden on my children' is a good example. Sometimes this sentiment conceals a 'selfish' wish to get a bit of peace and quiet after a lifetime of work, or a fear of being unwelcome. At other times, it can be taken at face value: the speaker means just what she says. It is the task of researchers and policy-makers to try to distinguish between these different possibilities, not on the basis of our own preconceptions, but by being as sensitive as possible to the nuances of what people say, and what lies behind their words.

In conclusion, we believe there are grounds for basing provision for older people in urban Mexico on the same principle as in Europe or the rest of North America: supporting people living independently in their own homes as long as possible. Networks of relatives and friends living close to each other provide a strong basis on which to build provision; but policy-makers should not automatically rely on the immediate family as the source of accommodation and care for tomorrow's older people.

Ann Varley is a Reader at the Department of Geography, University College, 26 Bedford Way, London WC1H 0AP, UK. E-mail: a.varley@geog.ucl.ac.uk

Maribel Blasco, who worked with Ann on this research project, is at Roskilde University, Denmark, where she is finishing her PhD on young people's experiences of schooling in Guadalajara.

Notes

1 *Gendered Housing: identity and independence in urban Mexico*, Economic and Social Research Council, UK, Research Grant R 000 23 6808.
2 This calculation is based on data from INEGI (1993). The 1990 census recorded 4,988,158 people of 60 years or more: 6.2 per cent of the national population.
3 Forty-five women of 60 or over expressed a preference.

References

Barer, B M (1994), 'Men and women aging differently', *International Journal of Aging and Human Development*, Vol. 38, No. 1, pp.29–40

Contreras de Lehr, E (1992), 'Aging and family support in Mexico', in Kendig, Hashimoto, and Coppard (eds) *Family Support for the Elderly: The International Experience*, Oxford University Press, New York, pp.215–23

de Vos, S (1990) 'Extended family living among older people in six Latin American countries', *Journal of Gerontology: Social Sciences*, Vol. 45, No. 3, pp.87–94

INEGI (Instituto Nacional de Estadística, Geografía e Informática) (1993), *La tercera edad en México*, INEGI, Aguascalientes

LeVine, S with Sunderland Correa, C (1993), *Dolor y alegría: Women and Social Change in Urban Mexico*, University of Wisconsin Press, Madison

Llera Lomelí, S R (1996), 'Gender Differentials in the Housing Conditions of the Mexican Elderly, 1970-1990', PhD Dissertation, University of Pennsylvania

Lloyd-Sherlock, P (1997), *Old Age and Urban Poverty in the Developing World: The Shanty Towns of Buenos Aires*, Macmillan, Basingstoke

López, M P and H Izazola (1994), *El perfil censal de los hogares y las familias en México*, INEGI, Aguascalientes

Montes de Oca, V (1999), 'Experiencia institucional y situación social de los ancianos en la ciudad de México', in Ziccardi and Cordera (eds), *Política social en México: decentralización, diseño y gestión*, Instituto de Investigaciones Sociales, UNAM, Mexico City

Tout, K (1989), *Ageing in Developing Countries*, HelpAge International and Oxford University Press, Oxford

Varley, A and Blasco, M (1999), '"Reaping what you sow"? Older women, housing and family dynamics in urban Mexico', in United Nations International Research and Training Institute for the Advancement of Women (INSTRAW) (ed.), *Ageing in a Gendered World: Women's Issues and Identities*, INSTRAW, Santo Domingo, 153–78

Transitions and boundaries:

research into the impact of paid work on young women's lives in Jordan

Mary Kawar

This paper explores the economic and social impact of the growing participation of young urban women in the workforce in Amman, Jordan. The writer argues that there is a new 'stage' in women's life-course in Jordan: single, employed adulthood. This is expanding young women's horizons, and challenging relationships between women and men, and between different generations, at all levels of society, including within the household. However, traditional values concerning family honour are challenged by this, and are sometimes being reinforced through new forms of control over young women.

This article is based on research that I undertook[1] into the current trend for young women in Amman, the capital of Jordan, to take up paid employment. I set out to explore how young women's employment affects – and is affected by – their relationships with their families, and how conventions about gender and age are challenged by this development.

Jordan, a small country in the Middle East, has enjoyed remarkable growth over the past 30 years. Reasons for this growth include its favourable geopolitical location during the oil boom in the neighbouring Arab Gulf Region in the 1970s. Jordanian skilled workers migrated to the Gulf countries and sent substantial remittances home as a result. In addition, Jordan has attracted substantial financial aid from oil-rich Arab countries (World Bank 1994). A related reason for economic growth is Jordan's quasi-liberal regime, which has aimed to foster stability – and hence investment – in a turbulent region of the world. Jordan has indirectly benefited in economic terms from two conflicts in the region: the civil war in Lebanon from the mid-1970s until the early

1990s, and the Iran–Iraq war of the 1980s. These conflicts prompted much business and private capital to relocate to Jordan, and, during the Iran–Iraq war, goods bound for land-locked Iraq passed through Aquaba port in Jordan.

However, Jordan's growth has been hampered by two economic 'shocks'. The first of these was the debt crisis, and the ensuing economic stabilisation policies of the late 1980s. During the 'oil boom' years, Jordan had accumulated billions of dollars in debt (Satloff 1992). The global recession of the late 1980s and early 1990s caused an economic crisis in oil-producing countries, and this had a knock-on effect for Jordan, reducing employment of migrant workers in the Gulf, and reducing financial aid to the government of Jordan from the Gulf States. In addition, Iraq's invasion of Kuwait in 1990 caused an alarming influx of an estimated 300,000 'returnee' migrant workers into Jordan. In 1988, Jordan unveiled a major austerity plan, including a 50 per cent devaluation of the Jordanian dinar, in addition to new duties and taxes to reduce the budget deficit.

Employment in Jordan

The economic crisis and subsequent adjustment has affected the Jordanian population in terms of inflation, and a deteriorating standard of living. It has been estimated that 23 per cent of the Jordanian population was living below the national poverty line in 1997 (El Solh 1999). Unemployment rates have increased dramatically. Unemployment has always affected women more adversely than men in the Arab region as more limited types of occupations are available for them (Economic Research Forum 1998; El-Solh 1999). In particular, a larger proportion of women is dependent on public-sector employment than is the case for men. In 1997, unemployment rates for women were 28.5 per cent, compared with 11.7 per cent for men (Department of Statistics 1999).

Despite this, the underlying trend of employment patterns in Jordan seems to be slow change in favour of women. Traditional stages in Jordanian women's lives are based on rigid hierarchies determined by gender and generation. Women start out as girl-children and mature into unmarried adolescents, dependent on their parents. Finally, they become dependent wives and mothers. Young women's opportunities in employment are expanding: despite low official rates of economic activity, women's employment almost doubled between 1979 and 1997, from 7.7 to 14 per cent of the female population, and the rate of growth of female employment exceeded the rate of growth of male employment (Economic Research Forum 1998). Other indicators of change that shape women's ability to gain employment and transform their lives more generally are, first, increasing levels of female education: illiteracy among women decreased from 48 per cent in 1979 to 20 per cent in 1996, while 47 per cent of those enrolling in tertiary education were women in 1997 (Department of Statistics

1999). Second, the average age of marriage has increased from 17 years in 1971 to almost 24 years in 1995 (ibid).

The research

Both quantitative and qualitative research tools were used, including a survey of 36 private-sector employers, and a questionnaire survey of women between 20 and 30 years old, in 302 households in Amman. The women were either working, unemployed, or economically inactive,[2] single, and not enrolled in education at the time of the interview. I visited 40 of the households again, to conduct more detailed semi-structured interviews. These were held with young women themselves, and, depending on household circumstances, with other family members as well.

In general, respondents came from large households, with an average of 7.9 members. Household income varied widely, but the average annual *per capita* income was US$963. The average educational attainment of respondents was quite high: 58 per cent had had post-secondary education, and 40 per cent of those who were employed worked in professional and technical occupations (most were teachers). Another 20 per cent worked in the manufacturing sector, followed by 15 per cent in clerical occupations. However, despite the high education levels and the tendency to work in professional occupations, average wages were quite low: 54 per cent of the sample earned less than US$140 per month.

Family perceptions of young women's employment

The desirability of education and employment

Higher education was regarded in a positive light by the families of women involved in the study (even if it means interacting with men, living away from home and so on). The women in the study are among the first generation to begin reaping the benefits of expanding female educational opportunities, and subsidised colleges and universities.

Among all income groups, higher education of daughters has become linked to prestige. However, women's families expect them to pursue studies that do not challenge traditional female gender roles, and this expectation shapes women's choices.

In the process of gaining higher education, young women are exposed to new ideas, different ways of life, and social freedom. Higher education nurtures ambition and creates aspirations for economic and social independence. These could be dampened by a lack of employment opportunities, but it seemed that, for women whom I interviewed, the experience of undertaking higher education had in itself changed their attitudes to, and expectations of, life.

Employment, on the other hand, is regarded by the young women's families as a potential threat to traditional norms of sex segregation. In cases where women have studied subjects in higher education that are considered unsuitable for women, families are particularly likely to place restrictions on their daughters' employment. Such restrictions might include telling young women to find work that enables them to work close to home, to work hours that will always allow them to reach home before dark, or to find single-sex working environments.

For example, one young woman was encouraged to pursue a government-sponsored youth-training scheme for mechanics, but later she was not allowed to seek employment. Her family considers that her skill could only be used in a 'male' job, which would be inappropriate for her. In such situations as these, parents tended to take pride in their daughters' achievements, despite the fact that they remain unemployed. In fact, the young mechanic was almost regarded as a hero within her household and neighbourhood, for symbolically breaking gender barriers. As soon they learned of my research topic, neighbours directed me to her house, explaining that she had managed to train for a man's job.

Sometimes, parents had a narrow view of educational attainment, and used this to justify restrictions on daughters' employment. For example, one young woman had a degree in finance. According to her parents, she could only aim to work in a bank, although she had many opportunities for work as an assistant accountant in private companies. This was prohibited by her parents, who see small firms as presenting potential risk to their daughter's reputation (see below).

Acceptable types and conditions of work

Having established that there is a disjointed relationship between educational attainment and subsequent employment for young women in Amman, we can now turn to the question of what parents see as acceptable work for their daughters, and why they think as they do. In the main, this hinges on notions that women and men should work segregated from each other, in a 'respectable' working environment. (Many, but not all, parents share these ideas: many women do work in mixed-sex environments.) One pre-dominant concern among many families is that a daughter should be home before dark. In general, women working as teachers do not face difficulties here, since school days are short. This provides another incentive for young women to enter teaching, in addition to the fact that teaching is considered a respectable female job. Some manufacturing industries accommodate the needs of women workers to get home before dark.

Another form of restriction placed on young women is the location of their workplaces. Social restrictions on women's movement, and the importance of women's good behaviour in public, mean that some parents do not allow their daughters to use public transport, because this is used mostly by men. However, young women reported that they have found solutions to this obstacle. For example, if there is a well-known employer, and several women from the same community begin work there, travel becomes acceptable, since young women can commute together daily. This serves many purposes: they can keep an eye on one another's behaviour; they tend not to be harassed by strangers, since they are in a group; and, because more than one woman commutes, it is hard for the community to disapprove of their employment in distant parts of the city.

Another form of parental restriction on daughters' employment is that the family should know the prospective employer. Thus, where possible, daughters work for relatives, family friends, or neighbours. If an employer happens to be unknown, the family will make inquiries about him; that is, try to ascertain his 'reputation' (mainly as regards his attitude to, and treatment of, women workers). When a young woman finds work, her father or brothers will want to meet the employer and finalise her conditions of employment face to face. A father will say to the employer: 'I am entrusting you with my daughter', and the employer answers: 'Do not worry. She will be like my own daughter as long as she is working here.'

In turn, I was told, the employers who depend on young female labour exercise two strategies to accommodate family restrictions on female mobility. First, employers can set up their business in proximity to labour supply, usually near congested low-income neighbourhoods, where women need to work. An example in Amman is the area of Hai Nazzal, which

has high rates of female employment in clothing and food-production enterprises. Most workshops were literally down the hill from this area. In the mornings and afternoons it is possible to see groups of young women walking to and from work together. The second strategy, used by large manufacturing employers, is to provide transportation for their women workers.

Many families find the working conditions unacceptable in employment in other kinds of establishments – specifically small ones in the private sector. Various reasons were given for this, including the fact that working hours are longer. In addition, unlike large establishments and public-sector employers (banks, the teaching professions, or manufacturers), employers do not provide concessions for female labour such as transport or daylight working hours. Finally, very few private-sector firms have sex-segregated work spaces.

Preventing sexual harassment at work

Many of the above restrictions put on the conditions of young women's work are means of preserving the sexual reputation of young women, and preventing sexual harassment. The term 'sexual harassment' – which tends to be seen as actual physical or verbal abuse – needs to be redefined in such a context. Women's reputations – and those of their families – are critical to their futures, and may be harmed by the threat of sexual harassment, or even by mere gossip.

From the research, it seems that both young women and their families perceive male employers in general to be potential threats to female workers' reputation. Consequently, any employer who needs female labour has to prove his innocence among the young women themselves, as well as to their families. One strategy that I encountered here was that an older woman (sometimes the wife of the employer) will work as the general supervisor in small workshops with exclusively female labour.

The preoccupation with keeping young women's sexual reputations intact has resulted in some cases in a rather rigid form of male-boss/female-worker relations in the workplace: employers need to act like fathers, and young women need to act like daughters, and it is necessary for young women and employers alike constantly to prove their innocence. This has been described as the 'de-sexualisation' of workplace communities, as men and women seek to de-emphasise the sexual connotations of their physical closeness in the workplace, and thus defuse the threat to their reputation (Kabeer 1995).

However, sometimes the idea of a 'father–daughter' relationship can allow employers to harass young women. One young woman told me:

'One day, my boss, whom I respect very much, touched my hand and then my hair. I screamed. He then said: "What's the matter? You are like my daughter." He never touched me again. I think he was testing how I would react, and my reaction made him treat me like a daughter. He takes care of me, and recently asked the management to give me a raise. All the other secretaries are jealous of me, and started rumours about me and my boss. He is a very good man, and when he was sick I visited him in hospital and gave him flowers. His wife does not like me.'

Young women who know very few men, apart from their own fathers and relatives, may find it hard to distinguish between harassment and filial relations. In addition, they may themselves become attracted to men whom they work with. (As in this particular case, this may take the form of innocent admiration or respect.) The fact that young women are conditioned to see themselves as the vulnerable sex means they may take measures to avoid harassment. For example, some young women claimed to me that they had refused employment opportunities because

they did not trust the boss or co-workers. Many of the young women interviewed knew of stories about unknown women who have been taken advantage of in unknown workplaces. There was no way of telling whether these accounts were fact or fiction.

It seems that young women's need to protect their sexual reputation reinforces their economic and psychological dependence on their families. It was a common belief among respondents that women in dire economic need are more exposed to harassment by employers. Some women interviewees expressed relief that their own families would never expose them to situations where their reputations might suffer, no matter what their economic needs.

Young women's views on employment

This section explores the perceptions of young women workers themselves. How do they perceive the existing gender division of labour in employment? What do they think of their experience of employment? How does it affect their perception of their role as daughters and siblings within the household? Finally, has going out to work given them more personal autonomy to determine their own paths in work and marriage?

Attitudes towards 'acceptable' female work

All young women respondents were asked to say what they thought were the three most suitable professions for women. A substantial number – 44 per cent – said they thought that women should work in professions consistent with their 'nature' as women. This particular attitude was similar among all women respondents, regardless of whether they were categorised as employed, unemployed, or inactive. Not surprisingly, 66 per cent of the sample survey thought that the most appropriate profession for a woman is teaching. The reasons given were that it is consistent with their roles as mothers. Also, 65 per cent of the sample survey thought that women should work in sewing and embroidery – an extension of women's 'natural' abilities in handiwork.

Such attitudes are not necessarily determined by what these young women think about female ability, but by the options that they perceive are available for women (Nawar et al 1995). Even those who believe that women can perform any kind of occupation would not necessarily take up the challenge of an unacceptable occupation. In assessing young women's attitudes towards the gender-typing of jobs, therefore, differences must be made between beliefs and actual behaviour.

What makes for work satisfaction?

Because of the various constraints placed on finding appropriate employment, very few women are in what they perceive to be 'unsatisfactory' working conditions. However, since most respondents who are working are employed in jobs that are conventional for women, the overwhelming compromise is accepting low pay: 17 per cent think they are underpaid. Despite this, women said they rarely demand rises in pay, since they know their working conditions are attractive to many other women. In finding appropriate working environments, they are effectively constrained from expanding their earning powers.

As far as personal fulfilment is concerned, it seems safe to say that very few young women in low-paid jobs in conventionally 'female' sectors experience much sense of achievement. The majority, who are in the manufacturing sector or the lower echelons of the services sector, said that they did not really enjoy their work. The greatest – and only – satisfaction is that they are able to move out of restrictive home environments, where they are bored, and establish social contacts. Most of them realise that there is a lack of future opportunities, but said that they do not aspire for more in any case.

Even the young women who are in professional occupations, and should therefore be able to establish a career, tend to be seen by employers and families in terms of conventional gender roles. Ambitious young women may be afraid to distance themselves from their female and male colleagues, and/or deter marriage prospects through unconventional behaviour. Ambitious and confident woman can be described in Arabic by employers and colleagues as *mistarjileh*. This has a double meaning: 'she is like a man', and 'she would rather be a man'. In other words, the aspirations that make an enthusiastic or efficient worker are considered to be masculine.

Young women professionals in non-segregated occupations reported trying to work hard and yet remain carefully 'feminine', avoiding being described as similar to men in their behaviour. This balance is achieved through working hard and securing employers' approval, while remaining generally undemanding and non-assertive. As one young woman architect explained:

'I am the only woman architect in our firm. Before my arrival the other women were the secretaries. I work the hardest and currently have the heaviest load. However, when we need to go to the site, my boss sends my male colleagues. He says the labourers on the construction sites will not take me seriously. When clients come, he never lets me sit in meetings, but male colleagues are usually invited in. For this he always has excuses, like he does not want to waste my precious time. I feel that if I want to continue with my current work, which I enjoy and which gives me a lot of responsibility, I need to undermine my achievement, especially in front of my male

colleagues. As for my boss, he does appreciate me and never stops praising me, but only when we are alone.'

Impact of earning income

Perhaps the most revealing assessment of the impact that earning income can have on young women's lives came from those with previous work experience, but who were unemployed at the time of the interview. Several such women stated that when they were income-earners they were more involved in family decisions, and felt that they were treated with more respect than their current situation. One young woman stated:

'These days, my brothers keep interfering in my life. They want to know where I go and who I see. When I used to work, things were different. They were hard up, and I used to loan them money. It gave me so much pleasure, because they could never interfere in my life and I even controlled their expenses. As soon as they tried to assume the big-brother role, I would threaten that I would not give them any more money. One day, as I was leaving to visit a friend, my brother wanted to know where I was going. I said: "Listen, one more question and you hand back every penny you owe me right now." Now, things have changed. It is they who are working and I am unemployed.'

However, there are also many young women who did not feel that earning income had any effect on their status within the household. Several even thought that they would be better off if they were not working. One stated:

'My mother expects me to do all the housework after my return from work. She thinks that since she always cared for us, now it's my turn to care for her. She does not realise that I am exhausted, and accuses me that I am lazy. All my father cares about is my money. One month I could not give him any and he screamed: "Damn you and your money."

He did not talk to me until I gave him money the following month. My married sisters continually expect me to loan them money and give them presents. When I don't, they accuse me of being stingy. Work has brought me nothing.'

In short, the impact of earning on the role and status of young women differs from household to household. Earning sometimes increases status, and at other times increases subjugation. The two conflicting case studies above are both based on low-income families where young women's pay is limited. In higher-income households, the dependence on daughters' wages is not an issue, and therefore does not pose threats to power relations – in particular, to the position of males.

Impact on personal autonomy

I asked about the issue of personal autonomy by focusing on two elements: first, the impact of work on physical mobility and social freedom, and second, young women's personal aspirations and whether they manage to fulfil them. However, the degree to which an individual can behave autonomously always depends on the specific or individual social context (Nawar et al 1995).

Mobility and social freedom

Physical freedom, in particular, is closely related to young women's psycho-social development as girls, irrespective of whether or not they are employed. Girls learn to fear being alone in certain places from a young age, and this, in effect, limits their confidence in being in public spheres as adults.

The young women in my research had different concepts of freedom of movement. One respondent defined it as being free to visit relatives, while for another it meant being able to travel abroad. With this in mind, I asked the young women to say whether they were free to go to various specific destinations – the market, the doctor's, to see friends, to see relatives, and to go abroad – and whether they had to be escorted or not.

Working women were more mobile than women defined as economically inactive. The degree of freedom of movement of working and unemployed women was similar. For example, when going to market, 76 of employed women and 72 per cent of unemployed women could go alone, compared with 49 per cent of economically inactive women. This suggests that freedom of movement may be expanded through the fact of having been employed at some point. It is likely that some women who cease to work can maintain the same amount of freedom that they had gained through their employment. However, there is a significant number of women, regardless of employment status, whose freedom of movement is dependent on being escorted by a family member or close friend. When going to the market, 22 per cent of employed women, 25 per cent of unemployed women, and 39 per cent of economically inactive women were escorted.

There is a general trepidation among many young women in Jordan about being on their own in public spaces. Young women may see themselves as vulnerable and liable to attract unwanted attention, so avoid venturing out on their own: not because they are prohibited from doing so, but because many lack the self-confidence to do so. As one young woman stated, *'When I am walking alone in the street, I feel everyone is watching me.'*

In general, respondents felt that the attitudes of parents who insist on their daughters being escorted are not a sign of distrust, but show concern about protecting their reputation and public image. Many parents feel that young women have the relative freedom to choose to go anywhere, as long as they are escorted.

Autonomy and personal aspirations

Studies of the impact of employment on women's lives have paid limited attention to personal aspirations. 'Despite a greater sensitivity to changing gender and other divisions of labour based on age and marital status within the household, attention to individual activities and aspirations frequently remain subsumed to a pre-occupation with the characteristics of the collective unit' (Sage 1993, 243).

Since the period between childhood and adulthood – youth itself – is traditionally 'squeezed out' of Arab women's life-courses, young women learn to suppress their personal hopes and aspirations, even if they continue, at a deep level, to long to realise them. Many hopes and aspirations relate to a desire to rise above the limitations on their social freedom and mobility.

'I used to be a basketball champion at school, and my teachers recommended that I join the national Jordanian team. My parents, of course, refused. Since finishing school, I have not played any sport. I have such an urge to exercise that sometimes I lock myself in my room and just jump till I am exhausted.'

In Jordan, the conventional physical and social restrictions imposed on young women deny them many forms of expression. These aspirations concern things they have been exposed to at school, on television, or, in the case of one woman who wanted to drive a car, on the street on a daily basis. Such aspirations are particular to their age group. Both fathers and mothers have had a different life experience, and are likely to misunderstand and consequently block their daughters' desires. Most young women understand this gap between themselves and their parents, and rarely attempt to challenge it, while being well aware of their predicament. In addition, they are usually left with no social confidence to challenge their parents. Employment gives many young women a route for self-expression, and breaks the monotony of restricted lives. For many, it represents a symbol of their desires to become independent adults.

Attitudes towards marriage and future gender roles

The concept of employment after marriage was acceptable to more employed and unemployed women than to women categorised as economically inactive. However, when attitudes towards employment after having children were explored, this difference in opinion narrowed. It seems that when assessing young women's attitudes towards work and marriage, the most meaningful distinction to be made is between a working wife and a working mother. A substantial number of employed women said that they would ideally like to stop work after having their first child. Even those who believed that women should not withdraw from the paid workforce as a result of motherhood qualified their view as follows: *'As long as a woman fulfils her duties as mother and wife, she should be able to continue with her work.'*

The idea that household chores should be redistributed between women and men was not in question: it was assumed that working mothers and wives have dual roles. Another group of women stated that work after marriage depends on 'family circumstances' – in other words, on financial need. These thought that a mother's employment is legitimate when it is for 'the family' or to 'help her husband'.

Despite these views, many respondents were also keen to discuss the importance of a wife's financial autonomy. This reveals that young women's experiences have exposed them to different ideas, and perhaps even empowered some of them to a degree, but they have also brought problems and dilemmas, chiefly regarding the question of living as single women in an overwhelmingly married society. As a result, young women may tend to downplay the importance of economic autonomy in order to fulfil their ascribed gender roles, even if they think it is important.

Conclusions

This article has investigated the changes in gender relations in Jordan, and the new boundaries that are being negotiated as a result of young women's later age of marriage, increasing education levels, and wider employment opportunities. This is a new stage in the life-courses of Jordanian women. Education and the possibility of employment have placed some young women in a position to balance taking up employment with conformity to conventional gender roles and relations. Although negotiating these changes is difficult and presents problems, some of the women interviewed seem to have started on a road to greater autonomy and personal fulfilment. One of the more important insights here is the complexity of the relationship between women's employment and the increased social and economic autonomy of women. The greatest changes for women are more likely to be effected within the home, rather than at a place of employment or through political change (Moore 1988). The centrality of the family in perpetuating unequal power relations between men and women cannot be overestimated.

Mary Kawar is the ILO's Specialist on Women Workers and Gender Questions, at the ILO Regional Office for Arab States, PO Box 11-4088, Beirut, Lebanon. Fax: 961-1-752406, e-mail: kawar@ilo.org. This article is based on a paper that was first delivered at a conference on 'Adolescent Girls' Livelihoods: Essential Questions, Essential Tools', at the Population Council, Cairo, 13–14 October 1999. The research was conducted before the author joined the ILO, and opinions expressed here do not necessarily reflect the views of the ILO.

Notes

1 My research was undertaken for a PhD degree completed in 1997.

2 I am using the standard ILO definition adopted in 1982. The unemployed are defined as those 'without work', 'currently available for work', or 'seeking work'. Work is assumed to be paid. I defined 'economically inactive' as those with no desire to work, rather than those who are simply not taking active steps to seek work. This is because many women in the context in Jordan (and in many other contexts) do not have the freedom to seek work, regardless of their desire, sometimes because they lack the access to formal channels to seek work. (For more on definitions of employment status or measurements of female labour-force participation, see Lim 1996, and Anker and Anker 1995).

References

Abu Lughud, L (1993), *Writing Women's Worlds: Bedouin Stories*, University of California Press, USA

Anker and Anker (1995), 'Measuring female labour force participation with emphasis on Egypt', in Khoury and Moghadam (eds): *Gender and Development in the Arab World*, Zed, UK

Department of Statistics (1999), *Women and Men in Jordan: A Statistical Portrait*, Department of Statistics, Amman, Jordan

Economic Research Forum (1998), 'Economic Trends in the MENA Region'. Website: http://erf.org.eg

El-Solh, C (1999), 'Gender Poverty and Employment in the Arab Region', paper presented at the Sub-Regional Planning Seminar on Gender Poverty and Employment for the Arab States, Beirut, Lebanon, 1–4 December 1999.

Kabeer, N (1994) *Reversed Realities: Gender Hierarchies in Development Thought*, Verso, UK

Kabeer, N (1995), *Necessary, Sufficient or Irrelevant? Wages and Intrahousehold Power Relations in Urban Bangladesh*, Working Paper 25, IDS, University of Sussex, UK

Kawar, M. (1997), 'Gender, Employment and Life Course: The Case of Working Daughters in Amman Jordan', unpublished PhD thesis, London School of Economics

Lin Lean Lim (1996), *More and Better Jobs for Women: An Action Guide*, International Labour Office, Switzerland

Moore, H (1988), *Feminism and Anthropology*, Polity Press, UK

Papps, Ivy (1993), 'Attitudes to female employment in four Middle Eastern countries', in Afshar (ed): *Women in the Middle East: Perceptions, Realities and Struggles for Liberation*, Macmillan Press, UK

Nawar, L, Lyod, C and Ibrahim, B (1995), 'Women's autonomy and gender roles in Egyptian families', in Makhlouf Obermeyer (ed): *Family, Gender and Population in the Middle East: Policies in Context*, American University of Cairo Press, Egypt

Sage, C (1993), 'Deconstructing the household: women's roles under commodity relations in highlands Bolivia', in Momsen and Kinnard (eds): Different Places, *Different Voices: Gender and Development in Africa, Asia and Latin America*, Routledge, UK

Satloff, R (1992), 'Jordan's great gamble: economics of crisis and political reform', in Barkey (ed), *The Politics of Reform in the Middle East*, St Martin's Press, USA

World Bank (1994), *Hashemite Kingdom of Jordan Poverty Assessment*, Vol. 1, report number 12675-JO, World Bank, USA

Community research on older women in the Dominican Republic

Jacquie Cheetham and Wendy Alba

This article looks at action-research into the interests and needs of older women in 11 urban communities in Santo Domingo, Dominican Republic. The research was instigated by Aquelarre (CEAPA), with help from International Co-operation for Development (ICD); Fundompromued (the Dominican Foundation for the Protection of Women of the Third Age); and informal women's groups. The findings of the research have become the basis of further community development work, which is being undertaken by the older women themselves.

The Dominican Republic (DR) is one of the Spanish-speaking Caribbean islands, with a population of 8 million (Centre of National Statistics), of whom approximately 2.5 million live in its capital, Santo Domingo. According to some international studies, about half of the country's population – some 3,300,000 people – live in poverty (*The World Guide* 1997/8, 30).

The DR was the first colony established in the Americas by Christopher Columbus in 1492. The DR has had a tumultuous history, beginning with the genocide of its indigenous population, the importation of African slaves from the start of the sixteenth century (which enabled the DR to become a major sugar-producing country), and later occupations by neighbouring Haiti, and the United States of America. The DR has been ruled by a number of powerful dictators, who have played a key role in suppressing the social, economic, and political development of the nation.[1]

However, today there is a thriving interest in politics among the population, which is relatively young, in common with many other Latin American countries:

34 per cent of the population is under 14 years (CIA 1999). However, there are growing government concerns, which are shared by NGOs working with older people, about the welfare of the DR's elderly. Currently, the official figure for the proportion of the population aged over 60 is 6 per cent, and it is estimated that this will grow to 14 per cent by 2030 (Centre of National Statistics). There is currently no social-security provision for older people, unless they have been employed as civil servants. Basic services including water, sanitation, and electricity supplies are inadequate: for example, only 59 per cent have access to safe drinking water (*The World Guide* 1997/8). The lack of State support, allied to the poor public health service, and year-round hot and humid weather conditions, leave many older people at risk of disease and illness.

Another factor that is important in understanding the situation of the elderly is changes in roles and attitudes with economic globalisation, growing urbanisation, and deepening poverty. There is a common conception in many 'developed' countries that the older people in poorer 'developing' countries are valued and respected as important community members, and have clear roles. However, this seems to be changing fast.

Working with older women

Since 1993, Aquelarre has been working in Santo Domingo, to end child abuse and violence against women in the home, promote good health among women, and the well-being of older women. Our anti-violence work is in partnership with other women's groups in DR, but ours was the only organisation in DR to focus specifically on older women as a target group. Aquelarre began working with older women as a separate socio-economic group in 1993, inviting them to join support groups and learning about the needs of the groups. Women in communities on the western fringe of Santo Domingo have formed community groups, while some women from 12 communities from eastern Santo Domingo formed their own organisation – Fundompromued – in July 1997.

Aquelarre has continued to work in partnership with Fundompromued, and, in 1998, the organisations began a joint study of the needs and priorities of older women in 11 communities in the north-east and north-west of the city (nine communities where Fundompromued had a presence, and two others where informal support groups had formed). The areas we focused on are densely populated, economically poor, and lack basic services. During the course of the research, participants identified a series of social problems in the areas, including insecurity, delinquency, drug abuse, disputes with neighbours, and lack of recreational spaces.

The research was informed by action-research principles.[2] Techniques included individual interviews with 70 older women, focus-group sessions with 120 women, and interviews with key community members.

The focus groups included some women aged below 55 who were interested in participating. The research was planned and implemented with the invaluable help of women community leaders, who acted as group co-ordinators, observers of the research process, and evaluators.

Problems and needs identified

Women were encouraged to identify their needs and problems, rank them in order of priority, and identify any solutions that they felt would resolve these problems. Most women identified health as their major concern, followed by economic issues and education. The fourth priority identified was 'family aspects': that is, their relationships with their families, family problems, and the needs of their children, grandchildren, and other relatives. (It should be noted that throughout the research there was a tendency for participants to focus on the needs of their loved ones, rather than their own needs and problems.)

Health

One of the principal rights with respect to older people defined by the United Nations with respect to older people specifies the right of maintaining health: 'Older people should have access to health care to help them maintain their optimal level of physical, mental and emotional health and to prevent deterioration and the commencement of illness' (UN Principles for Older Persons, Article 11).

When they were discussing health, older women seemed to be most comfortable about identifying their own personal needs, rather than focusing only on the needs of their families or communities. 85 per cent of those involved in the research identified health as their number-one personal priority. Two representative comments were: *'Health is the most important'* and *'... without health there is nothing'*.

Many conceptualise old age as a stage of life where people suffer a physical and mental deterioration. While the physical changes associated with the ageing process are visible to all, good health requires both emotional and physical well-being. When we asked key community members what they considered to be old age, a large proportion replied that they viewed ' old age' not only as the number of years that a person has lived, but also as an attitude or emotional state. It was pointed out that old age is usually seen as a negative stage of life. It is equated with a lack of energy, illness, lack of desire to do things, lack of vision, serious and conservative behaviour, and so on. Older women all too often internalise such myths and stereotypes about themselves, which are common in many contexts. Some older women in the research used phrases like *'I am like a girl of 16'* in a positive way, implying that it is a good thing for an older woman to behave as if she is younger. The women who used such phrases said they mean that they are energetic, fun-loving, and happy.

Such stereotypes are very misleading. The emotional problems of weakness and lack of physical energy are not solely experienced by older people. Not all young people have the positive attributes listed above; rather, some people are challenged by depression, lack of energy, or illness throughout their lives. In the words of one of the women in the research, *'lack of strength ... this is my problem from birth'*. In contrast, the majority of the older women with whom we work do not experience old age as a stage of either emotional or mental deterioration. On the contrary, they are active, keen to work and plan strategies to improve their lives and resolve their problems, and preoccupied as much with the future of their communities as with their own future or that of their families. It is ironic that such points need to be made, bearing in mind 'the number of older people leading the governments and institutions of the world' (Garrett 1993, 99.)

While the majority of older people maintain their mental abilities, it is of course possible that health problems can arise in older people. The women involved in the action-research felt that good health and adequate health care were essential to their enjoyment of their lives as older women. They discussed their physical health problems, the lack of public health services, and the prohibitively high cost of private heath provision. Lack of basic services was seen as a major problem for all involved in the research – older women and other community members alike. The older women pointed out that the lack of water and electricity in the areas where they live often results in more work for them, and in health problems. If services could be provided, life would change dramatically.

There are few specialist health facilities for older people in the DR, and little education on the health needs of older people. In our research, many older women discussed mental health problems in relation to the impact of poverty, social isolation, and family difficulties. It is clear that health services need to be holistic in their approach, and social services need to be developed alongside medical ones, in order to facilitate a healthy old age. Some health problems associated with ageing are caused by physical problems, and others by social difficulties. The majority of these may be temporary and could be reversed with treatment, but others may be permanent, and it is very important to distinguish between problems that can be treated, such as depression, and more permanent problems which do not have a known treatment at this stage, such as dementia, in order to treat people appropriately (Garrett 1993, 99). It is not uncommon for treatable health problems to be overlooked, while dementia is assumed to be the problem (ibid). Health professionals need to be educated and sensitised to these issues, and not rely on myths and stereotypes to inform their decisions.

Economic issues

Women do not only suffer discrimination in their older age, but have lived through 'years of disadvantageous positioning in the labour market and the pervasive discrimination that women encounter throughout their lives in schooling, work and housing. As a consequence, many women find themselves in poverty after retirement' (39th Session Report of the CSW).[3]

This general statement is borne out by the research findings, which confirm that many older women in Santo Domingo lack sufficient money to cover even their basic necessities. The women talked extensively about their vulnerable economic position. Typical comments included: *'We are hungry and we have no money.'* ... *'There is a lot of poverty ... At 11 or 12 in the morning ... the children have not eaten – a lot of older people have great needs.'* ...*'There is no money. I have six children, and I need to work to support the family.'*

Forty-seven per cent of the older women involved in the research are heads of households, 36 per cent are in households headed by their spouse, 9 per cent in households headed by their children, and the remaining 9 per cent are in other household formations. Eighty-nine per cent of the households that women formed a part of also included their children or grandchildren, nieces or nephews.

Only 5.7 per cent of the women in the study receive a State pension: the money that they receive is, in any case, very meagre: not enough to live on for a week, let alone a month. In many developing countries where there are little or no social-security provisions for people in old age,

governments claim that the responsibility of caring for older people lies with their families. This response not only ignores the needs of older people who do not have a family, but also denies older people their independence. Forty-seven per cent of the participants survive (completely or partly) on money that their children give them. Sixty-one per cent said that they lived with their families, and many of them reported that this was chiefly for economic reasons. Many told us that they found it very difficult to be economically dependent on their families, and said that they would like to achieve more independence through work, if they were able to get jobs. One woman told us that she needs work *'of an independent nature, so that I wouldn't have to be depending on the family'.*

Forty per cent said that their primary income is self-generated. On-going discrimination against older women in the labour market leaves them few opportunities to change this situation. Some women in our research had encountered discrimination against them in large-scale industrial employment. *'Sometimes they don't let you work (in the industrial free-trade zones) because you are old ..., because they don't want you'.* There is high unemployment in the Dominican Republic in general, but the women suggested that there should be places where older people could work: *'We need a zone for older people, a zone of work, something for us to do'.*

Discrimination also exists both in private-sector businesses and in private houses that employ domestic workers. One participant told us: *'For an older person, if they want to work, there is almost nowhere ... they don't even want an older woman to work in the house ...'* (Villa Esfuerzo, Los Solares). Another said: *'It is not easy – they don't want an old woman, because they say they don't want to bring death into the house.'* In all, only 16 per cent of the women in our research said that they worked outside the home for money.

Twenty-four per cent of the participants showed great resourcefulness in eking out a living through selling their services and working from home, in mainly traditional female roles: 13 per cent said they wash, cook, or sell food items and other things from home for money; 11 per cent said that they get paid for caring for children or other people, from their own or other families.

Economic necessity apart, many older people still wish to work, and continue contributing in a multitude of ways, using skills that they have developed over years. The women in the research stated very clearly that they wanted to work not only for economic reasons, but also from a desire to feel useful and active in the community, acknowledging the fact that work and self-esteem are intertwined. Women said they were proud of the work that they had done in their lives, and proud that they still had the ability and strength to work. *'I feel proud: I am 68 and have done a lot of work.' 'I have the desire and energy to work like any other.'*

Throughout the world, older women undertake long hours of unremunerated work within the home. Eighty-three per cent of the women in the research said that most of their time is spent in household chores. Forty-nine per cent said they spend a lot of time caring for their grandchildren, but only 11 per cent are paid for this work. Throughout the life-course, women's unpaid work in the home goes largely unrecognised by policy-makers, and is often not appreciated by the community. However, it is a great support to the family.

In the DR, as in other areas of the world, the work of older women provides the opportunity for the mothers and fathers of young children to work outside the home without the worry of child-care. 'Older women are not the passive consumers of benefits sustained by the efforts of a younger workforce. They are productive in old age, not only because

they support themselves, or free others to work, but because they contribute to the wellbeing and development of their community. Even those who are vulnerable and in need of economic and social support can play a part in shaping the future by sharing their past experience with the younger generations' (Payne 1995).

Education

While education is often associated with children and young people only, women in the study did not only stress its importance for their children and grandchildren, but they identified it as a need they face themselves. The desire for education is fuelled by the belief that with education one can improve life, both economically and emotionally. Sixty-eight per cent of those interviewed[4] said that they could read and write, compared with an overall literacy rate in the DR of 82 per cent. However, among those who said they could read and/or write, we observed many having significant difficulty doing so, beyond writing a few words or their names. Because of this, it was often difficult to find a scribe to record the small-group activities.

Many women said that they wanted to strengthen their literacy skills. They challenged their exclusion from educational opportunities, and were very keen to become involved in workshops and courses in order to learn: *'We want to educate ourselves, to pass our old age learning to be useful or more useful'*. The women said they needed an opportunity to learn alongside each other as older women, a curriculum focusing on the topics and themes that they are interested in, transport to educational facilities, financial support to pay for education, and understanding of any limitations on grounds of health and other commitments.

Women also said that they were keen to be education providers as well: *'Those that know something can teach others, although it may not be the quality of a teacher'* While some women were keen to teach children, others wanted to teach other women, and exchange their knowledge with others.

'Family aspects'

As stated earlier, women in the research selected 'family aspects' (relationships with their family) as the fourth most pressing issue facing them. During the course of the research, we saw that the women were always thinking of their families and the problems of their family members. We constantly reminded them to think of the issues that they themselves faced, and that were experienced by older women in general. However, this was difficult. For example, women did not tend to look at their own economic poverty in isolation from that of their families. Because their communities are very poor, the issue of family survival colours women's attitudes to many of the issues facing them as individuals. The women emphasised that if they had more money, they would be able to solve many of their family problems.

The experience of migration shapes older women's roles and status in family and community. The majority of older women in the research – including 90 per cent of the women who completed the individual questionnaires – had migrated from a rural area to Santo Domingo earlier in their life-course. These moves had usually occurred for family and economic reasons. Women in our research said they believed that if they still lived in rural areas, they would have retained traditional roles as advisers to younger people, and would have been respected figures in the community. Organisations representing the interests of older people, including HelpAge International, have argued that these roles within the community contribute to the preservation of older people's dignity and well-being and ultimately to their health (Garret 1993).

In contrast to the role of adviser, which many have lost, women in these Santo Domingo communities do retain a very active *practical* role, as carers for their grandchildren. Although many women were enthusiastic about this role, some pointed out that they lacked the physical and mental strength to bring up a second generation of children. Typical comments were: *'They leave the children here a lot, and it distresses me too much, to the point that I feel bad from the tension.'* Another said: *'In part I feel good, because I have become accustomed to the children, but sometimes I get too desperate … I don't know what to do with them. It makes me want to cry, the way they make me feel.'* Discussions at the focus-group sessions about the difficulties of being a grandmother highlighted the fact that often there is no private or personal space for them within the house.

Caring for grandchildren limits older women's options and independence. This was clear during the course of the research, when we found that it was often very difficult for women to attend meetings with us; some partly solved the problem by bringing their grandchildren with them. Many women expressed discontent with their families for having such expectations of them and putting pressure on them in this way.

The treatment of older people obviously varies between families, but there was widespread recognition of the maltreatment of older women in the family, and in society in general. One woman stated: *'They don't give you care, they don't give you affection, don't pay attention to the opinions of older people and have a lack of affection to the older people'.* This, she admitted, is *'not in all cases, but it happens'.*

The perception that there is a lack of respect for the older women from their children and grandchildren was also mentioned frequently. *'I have a son who doesn't respect me. I am tired of talking and not being listened to.'*

Solutions identified by participants

The second stage of the action-research was to encourage participants to identify practical solutions to their problems. First, they identified possible solutions available to individuals. These included 'the help of other people', 'co-operation', 'self-help', and 'divine power'. Next, they identified solutions available to a group of people. These included a striking acknowledgement of the power of group work as a motivator for participation and self-improvement, summed up in the words of one participant: *'If we are all together we have force, and being together, accompanying each other – in this way we can gain anything.'*

The women then discussed where they thought they could find help for these problems. Naturally, some groups in particular areas of the city were more aware than others of the resources and networks available. In all, women identified public bodies responsible for different services, including public health services, the town hall, the police, syndicates, the Institute of the Family (a government body), the Secretary of Education, and other officials and departments of the State. They also identified private businesses and neighbourhood groups. Other solutions identified included 'the government in general', the President, and God.

As part of the action-research process, all the different groups met each other and shared the results of the research; in this way, they were able to learn from each other about what was available to them.

Results of the action-research

Like many centres of its kind in both developing and developed countries, Aquelarre suffers from a constant shortage of funds and threats of funding cuts: at present, it is operating with three permanent and one temporary full-time members of staff. Despite these constraints, the energy and commitment of the older women who participated in our action-research is inspiring for us to witness.

Participants in the action-research have now selected a group of over 20 women from over 15 communities as community representatives. Despite the large distances between the communities in the north-east and north-west of the city that participated in the research, and the difficult transport conditions, which mean that a journey from west to east takes between one and two hours, women are now meeting monthly or bi-monthly to share the experiences from their work. They report that they are a constant source of inspiration and encouragement to each other.

The community representatives are currently being trained as *multiplicadoras* (community educators, trainers, and facilitators), by project workers from Aquelarre's new project, 'Gender and the Third Age'. This project was started as a result of the research. Both of us have contributed to training sessions, along with other local educators. The women themselves have selected the topics and areas that they consider as priorities for training. They then reproduce training sessions in their communities, and pass on what they have learned.

Fundompromued, Aquelarre's partner in the action-research, has received a small grant from the National Lottery Fund of the UK, through the Committee for a Dignified Old Age (an alliance of local government and NGOs working together to lobby the central government), and HelpAge International. Fundompromued has used the grant to purchase machinery and materials to begin training courses in the production of dolls, table-cloths, and household goods. Subsequently, it has begun to sell its products locally on a small scale. It has also managed to get an agreement with a local doctor to run a small health clinic once a week for the older women in north-eastern Santo Domingo. It is presently trying to raise enough capital to purchase a flat to use as premises for its activities, and to enable it to provide services. All these activities have developed as a result of the issues raised as priorities during the action-research.

The other two community groups involved in the research have also received a small grant from the UK Lottery Small Grants Fund, to open a Community Centre for Older Women: this will be the first in the country. Here, services offered will include weekly exercise classes, health services, educational and literacy classes, a support group, and a small coffee shop. An integral part of the work of establishing the Centre is developing a plan for how to make the centre self-sustainable after the funds have ceased in a year's time.

During the action-research, participants frequently emphasised that they needed solutions now to address poverty and lack of services: they have therefore prioritised the activities outlined above. At the same time, they are involved in other activities, including participating in talks and interviews with the local media, and holding activities in their communities to change the perception of older people and to promote intergenerational mixing. The women in each of the communities are involved in the activities of *Red por Una Vejez Digna* (Network for a Dignified Old Age), an alliance of local government and NGOs, working together to lobby the government.

In September 1998, the Network celebrated the result of its work: new legislation on the rights of older people in the Dominican Republic. The Law for the Protection of Older People (No. 352–98) is a great step forward in favour of older people in the DR. The Network must now lobby the government to comply with the law, which guarantees rights and services to older people, including a system of social security.

Jacquie Cheetham(jacquie_cheetham@ hotmail.com) and Wendy Alba (ceapa@aacr.net) work for El Centro de Apoyo Aquelarre.

Notes

1 For more background information on the Dominican Republic, see *The World Guide* 1997/8, and Ferguson 1992.
2 For further information on these principles, see Pretty et al., 1995.
3 Point 110, p.54.
4 We tried to collect statistical information of this nature in individual interviews.

References

Alba, W and Cheetham, J (1999), 'Diagnostic Comunitaio con mujeres maoyres'; CEAPA, Dominican Republic (unpublished as yet)

CIA (1999) *The World Fact Book* http://www.odci.gov/cia/publication/factbook/

Ferguson, J (1992), *The Dominican Republic: Beyond the Lighthouse*, Latin America Bureau, UK

Garrett, Gill (1993), *Adding Health to Years: a basic handbook on older people's health*, HelpAge International

HelpAge International – http:www.helpage.org

Payne, K (1995), ' Shaping the future – the contribution of older women' in Sharman (ed.), *Older Women in Development*, HelpAge International, UK

Pretty, J, Guijt, I, Thompson, J, and Scoones, I. (1995), *A Trainer's Guide for Participatory Learning and Action*, International Institute for Environment and Development (IIED) Participatory Methodology Series, Russell Press, UK

The World Guide 1997/8, CD-ROM, Hillco Media Group, Storgatan, Sweden

Girl-trafficking, HIV/AIDS, and the position of women in Nepal

Pratima Poudel and Jenny Carryer

This article focuses on trafficking of young Nepalese girls and women. Trafficking is an integral part of the social and economic fabric of Nepal, as in other parts of the world. The practice causes intolerable degradation and suffering for the girls and young women involved, who are treated as a commodity. It presents a risk to their physical and mental health, and in particular to their sexual health. The article examines the connections between coercive sex work and HIV infection, and community and government responses to HIV infection among trafficked sex workers. In particular, it considers the current AIDS prevention and control programme in Nepal, and criticises it from the feminist perspective of the authors, who are a Nepalese nurse who has undertaken academic work in New Zealand related to women's health, and a New Zealand feminist academic, who is also a nurse.

At present, very high numbers of young girls are being taken across Nepal's borders, as trafficked sex workers, to destinations that include India. The number of girls being trafficked to India is estimated to be 5,000–7,000 per year, with 20 per cent of them aged under 16 (Thapa 1997). Trafficking causes immense suffering to individual girls and women, and as such should be of extreme concern to all human-rights activists, governments, and non-government organisations (NGOs) concerned with human development. It is widely acknowledged at international level to be a serious violation of human rights, both internationally and in Nepal itself. In 1949, the United Nations passed a Convention for the Suppression of the Traffic in Persons and of the Exploitation of the Prostitution of Others. Nepal is a signatory to this, which should logically lead to a commitment to prosecute traffickers.

The trafficking of girls and women for prostitution is publicly recognised in Nepal to be a social evil: this is reflected in legislation against it, for example New Muluki Ain (1963), the Human Trafficking Control Act (1987), and the Special Provisions of Human Trafficking Act (1996). These laws impose penalties of 5–20 years for trafficking, depending on the level of involvement. However, trafficked girls and women are mostly illiterate and poor, and are therefore very unlikely to be able to fight against trafficking in a court of law. If someone decides to file a case, the slow pace of investigative and judicial processes and constant political intervention discourage her from fighting to the end. Another discouraging fact is that the State does not provide protection for witnesses.

The trafficking of girls and young women in Nepal has its roots in gender politics and sexual inequalities, linked to widespread economic poverty. Nepal is one of the poorest countries in the world, with a gross domestic product (GDP) of US$1137 (CIA 1999). About 85 per cent of the population live in the rural areas, and agriculture is the main source of livelihoods. Nearly half of Nepal's population lives below the poverty line. The level of educational attainment is very low, with one-third of males and two-thirds of females having never attended schools in rural areas (Ministry of Health/ New Era/DHS 1997)

The Constitution of the Kingdom of Nepal (1990) states that 'all citizens shall be equal before the law ... No discrimination shall be made against any citizen in the application of general laws on grounds of religion, race, sex, tribe or ideological conviction or any of these'. Despite this principle, discrimination against women starts at birth, with differing ways of rearing a girl and boy child. Education for girls is often regarded as a wasted investment, as girls will leave the family eventually, tradition demanding that every girl be married. About two-thirds of children of primary-school age (6–10 years) who are not enrolled are girls (NESAC 1998). There is a strong relationship between female education and age at first marriage: women marry on average at the ages of 16, 16.9, and 19.8 years, depending respectively on whether they have had no formal education, primary education only, or secondary schooling (Ministry of Health/ New Era/DHS 1997). Women's participation in politics is negligible, despite a 5 per cent reservation for female candidates in parliamentary and local government elections.

The people who deliver young girls and women into the hands of brokers are generally people in whom the girls have placed their trust, and this shows the degree to which such practices are covertly accepted. As late as 1951, there was a custom in Nepal of selling or presenting beautiful girls to the palaces, to serve as concubines and maids. This 'trafficking' may have ceased, but a new form – cross-border trafficking – has taken its place (Pradhan 1996). Most of the girls and women currently trafficked to India and other destinations are abducted by traffickers, having been sold by their own next-of-kin, parents, relatives of their husbands, or 'friends of the family' (O'Dea 1993). Some brokers arrange sham marriages for girls, or promise employment in Nepal or in foreign countries, and then sell them to brothels. Others may stage a rape, after which the girl is obliged to enter enforced prostitution. Some groups of brokers kidnap girls, then sell them at auction (Ghimire 1996, O'Dea 1993). Nepalese politicians are themselves involved in this 'business', and this reduces the efficiency of government agencies and non-government organisations who attempt to promote and enact policies to control the practice (Pradhan 1996).

Attitudes to HIV-positive trafficked women

Recently, the new disease of HIV/AIDS has increased the suffering caused by trafficking for both individual abused women, and for the wider society. HIV/AIDS and other sexually transmitted diseases are now prevalent across the urban and rural sectors of Nepal. In 1995, the World Health Organisation estimated 26,000 HIV-positive adults and children, at the adult infection rate of 0.24 per cent (WHO/UNAIDS 1997). These diseases are spread through sexual transmission, including heterosexual sex, which occurs within many different contexts, including commercial sex; and through other means, including drug abuse.

The main source of AIDS transmission in Nepal is heterosexual contact (Gurubacharya 1997). Currently, there are increasing numbers of young Nepalese girls living within Nepal, having been returned home by Indian brothel-keepers. Usually, the owners or the operators of brothels return women and girls to Nepal when they are suspected of having AIDS (Maiti Nepal 1997). In the mid-1990s, there were about 13,500 very young Nepalese girls in Bombay alone who were HIV-positive (Dixit 1996). In November 1998, Nepal's National Centre for AIDS and STD Control reported 1,175 HIV/AIDS cases, whereas unofficial estimates claim that there are 20,000–25,000 infected Nepalese (Maiti Nepal 1997). According to them, 60–70 per cent of the prostitutes returning from India carry HIV or other STDs. There are no reliable figures, mainly due to under-reporting and unrecognised cases.

The medical and social needs of those returning to Nepal, in such circumstances, are considerable. These women need medical services for physical treatment, they need emotional and counselling support, and they need to maintain confidentiality (Suvedi 1997). However, there is widespread ignorance and prejudice about HIV/AIDS-related illness and death in Nepal. HIV-positive ex-prostitutes are usually rejected by their families, as well as ostracised by the wider society. These attitudes are perpetuated by a very low literacy rate in rural areas, as discussed above. If the HIV-positive status of ex-sex workers comes to the attention of the police, they may be subjected to physical and mental torture, enforced medical examinations, and public exposure, often in the media, which will result in their being stigmatised for the remainder of their lives (Ghimire 1996).

Even if ex-sex workers can avoid such treatment on re-entering Nepal, they have few alternatives for survival. There is very little support from development policy or practice, whether governmental or non-governmental, for women who have been trafficked and return to Nepal. Skills-development programmes started by the Ministry of Social Welfare for the general population are insufficient to meet the level of need (ibid). The State has not established rehabilitation centres for such returnees, although in the current context this may not be desirable or effective. Many young girls and women who still have good health return to making money through sex work, facilitating the continuing transmission of HIV infection.

Some national and international NGOs, including Maiti Nepal, ABC Nepal, and CWIN, are currently active in the prevention of girl-trafficking and in the rehabilitation of trafficked girls. They provide the returnees with food and shelter, psychological treatment, medical treatment, legal support, and non-formal education like training in basic literacy, tailoring, weaving, and fabric-painting.

The AIDS prevention and control programme: a critique

In co-ordination with NGOs, the AIDS prevention and control units of the government of Nepal have undertaken several activities since 1995 (Gurubacharya 1997). The AIDS-prevention programme, formalised in 1996, has focused on provision of information. A campaign has been carried out, using electronic media, including radio and television, and face-to-face dialogues, via workshops and seminars. In addition, the prevention programme has included surveillance of the regions of the country (in particular, the Kathmandu valley), where trafficking and sex work is prevalent. This is carried out by social workers, and supported by NGOs. Outreach clinics give health education and offer condoms. People suffering from AIDS-related illnesses are referred to other health providers for treatment.

The way in which sexuality is understood in a society determines the measures that it decides to take to prevent sexually transmitted diseases, including HIV/AIDS. In Nepalese society, sexual relations are only understood as heterosexual encounters, and all other forms of sex are deemed illegal, as well as culturally unacceptable. Many women are confused by the contrast between their experience of sex and their expectations of romance, love, and caring. In Pratima Poudel's experience, women are expected to be virginal and modest about sexual matters, in tune with Hindu culture and tradition, and to rely on their husbands for sexual knowledge and direction. This is confirmed by research from development organisations (UNICEF 1996). The control that women can exercise over the safety of their sexual practices is constrained by these expectations.

In light of the above, it is surprising that women have been the principal target of Nepal's AIDS-prevention programme, and that the programme has concentrated on public education campaigns, which focus on condom-use to make sex safer.

Targeting women

Focusing exclusively on women implies that young girls and women are able to control the sexual encounter. This fails to take into account the realities of unequal power relations between women and men. The negotiation of safer sex in heterosexual encounters is shaped by the power that men can exercise over women at all levels in male-dominated societies, which interlinks with other power relations, including those determined by age, class, and ethnicity (Holland et al 1990). Young women and adolescent girls are even less likely to be able to negotiate with their partners than older women, since they also face unequal power relations between younger and older people.

Inequality between women and men in Nepal, which extends to inequality in negotiating sex, is reinforced by culturally based ideas of male dominance and strength, and female submissiveness. Traditional role expectations for women are to be passive, obedient, and self-sacrificing in relationships with their partners. There are no rights for women, and they have to maintain silence. Male control over female sexuality is a crucial mechanism for men to use to maintain their social and economic dominance over women, and male violence against women is an important instrument in maintaining that control. Sex workers, and in particular those young girls who have been coerced or trafficked, stand almost no chance of negotiating the nature of the sexual encounter, and protecting themselves. Thus, the AIDS-prevention programme fails to discuss unequal power relations between women and men in intimate relationships, and does not target men as traffickers and clients of trafficked girls and other sex workers.

Focusing on condoms

Public education about AIDS has a tendency to present sexual encounters as a set of acts leading up to penetrative intercourse, necessitating a condom for protection. This simplistic understanding of sex makes the process of prevention seem easier: simply a matter of timely intervention (Holland et al 1990, Zierler and Krieger 1998).

Young girls who have been trafficked are least likely to be able to negotiate such safer sexual practices, because they have been stripped of control over their own bodies. There is much evidence that condom use is not welcomed among men who have multiple sexual partners, including the clients of sex workers, and sex workers are not in a position to insist (Lear 1995, Zierler and Krieger 1998).

Even for women in non-coercive relationships, stressing condom use is an inadequate measure to prevent HIV infection. Women who can achieve safer sex by using condoms with one partner cannot necessarily negotiate their continued use as the relationship progresses, nor ensure that they can be used with subsequent partners. In addition, married women in many different contexts find it impossible to require their partners to use a condom on the grounds that they may have acquired HIV infection outside the marital relationship. Women attempting to introduce the subject of condoms in the context of such relationships risk appearing unfaithful, over-dominant, or inappropriately interested in sex (Poudel, personal observation in the trafficking-affected region of Sindhupalchowk, 1995).

Possible solutions

It is all too easy to engage in an academic critique of this situation, as we have done here. It is much more challenging to develop concrete means whereby the safety and quality of life for Nepalese girls – particularly those who are sold or otherwise coerced into sex work – is substantially improved. This short article has tried to address the issue of trafficking in women in relation to HIV/AIDS prevention strategies, rather than looking at the two issues in isolation. Government and NGO policy-makers also need to make these links. A holistic strategy is needed, to end trafficking, control HIV infection, and care for survivors of trafficking and for people living with AIDS. Such a strategy should be based on an understanding of gender inequalities in social and economic policies, the legal system, and education, and of discriminatory cultural practices. Only once these are transformed can real change take place in Nepal (Tuladhar 1996).

To eliminate the beliefs and practices that either actively support or ignore trafficking within Nepalese society, a very strong and multifaceted commitment is needed. National, regional, and international legislation is needed, to combat trafficking itself. Since the trafficking of young girls for sex work is a cross-border problem, and existing legislation is not effective, it is important for the Nepal government, in partnership with other governments of countries of the region, to review and improve existing legislation addressing trafficking for sexual exploitation and prostitution. Co-operative work is needed to develop a set of coherent and compatible laws and policies to eradicate trafficking and prostitution from both sides of national borders.

Nepalese public-health policies focusing on preventive measures to control the spread of AIDS must take account of the reality of inequality between women and men, which cross-cuts with age-based and economic inequalities to render young girls living in poverty vulnerable to sexual exploitation. Public education to combat the spread of HIV/AIDS should use an analysis of gender relations to increase public understanding of the ways in which it is contracted. In particular, there must be raised awareness of the way in which economic desperation and unequal power between women and men allow young girls' bodies to become a commodity for sale as an alternative to other sources of income. Newspapers and other media must contribute by disseminating information on the causes of trafficking, and the nature, prevention, and control of HIV infection, rather than sensationalising information about victims of sexual exploitation.

Current public-health campaigns to combat HIV/AIDS tend to expect women to take the responsibility not only for their own reputations and their own bodies, but also for policing men's sexual behaviour. Policy-makers must take responsibility for challenging male behaviour and changing it. If public-health campaigns are to be successful in reducing the heterosexual spread of HIV, then they must address the complex power relations in sexual encounters, which are shaped by gender, age, poverty, and other social factors. Health education should generate awareness of the sexual roles and responsibilities of men as well as women, stress the exploitative contexts in which women have sex with men, and give value to a wider range of safer sex practices, beyond condom use in situations of penetrative sex. They need, rather, to increase public awareness of more diverse forms of sexual expression, and create an opportunity for young girls and boys to understand and speak about sexuality in less limiting ways, before embarking on sexual relationships of their own.

Finally, communities, community-based organisations, NGOs, and government must respond at a local level to develop adequate support services for rehabilitation of victims and survivors of sexual exploitation. Above all, the punishment meted out to survivors – social marginalisation and continued economic deprivation – must cease.

Pratima Poudel is a registered nurse, now in clinical practice in Auckland: 2/33 Opaheke Road, Papakura, Auckland 1703, New Zealand. Email: ppoudel@yahoo.com

Jenny Carryer is Professor of Nursing at Massey University and Mid Central Health: Massey University, Private Bag 11222, Palmerston North, New Zealand. Email: J.B.Carryer@massey.ac.nz

References

ABC/Nepal (1996), NGO Report (3rd edition), *Red Light Traffic: The Trade in Nepali Girls*, Kathmandu, Nepal

CIA (1999) *The World Fact Book*, http://www.cia.gov/cia/publications/factbook/np.html

Dixit, S B (1996), 'Impact of HIV/AIDS in Nepal' in ABC/Nepal 1996

Ghimire, D (1996), 'Girl trafficking in Nepal – a situation analysis', in ABC/Nepal 1996

Gurubacharya, V L (1996) 'HIV/AIDS – everybody's concern', in ABC/Nepal 1996

Holland, J, Ramazonoglu, C, Scott, S, Sharpe, S and Thomson, R (1990), 'Sex, gender and power: young women's sexuality in the shadow of AIDS', *Sociology of Health and Illness*, Vol. 12, No.3, pp.336–50

Lear, D (1995), 'Sexual communication in the age of AIDS: the construction of risk and trust among young adults', *Social Science and Medicine*, Vol. 41, No. 9, pp.1311–23

Maiti Nepal (1997), 'Report on Cross-Border Workshop on Girl Trafficking', Birtamod, Jhapa, Kathmandu, unpublished.

NESAC (Nepal South Asia Centre) (1998), *Nepal Human Development Report 1998*, Nepal South Asia Centre, Nepal

Ministry of Health/ New Era/DHS (1997), *Family Health Survey 1996*, Macro International Inc, USA

O'Dea, P (1993), *Gender Exploitation and Violence: The Market in Women, Girls and Sex in Nepal*, UNICEF, Nepal

Pradhan, G (1996), 'The road to Bombay: forgotten women (Maya and Parbati, the end of dream)', in ABC/Nepal 1996

Suvedi, B K (1997), 'Ethics in relation to HIV/AIDS in Nepalese context', *Journal of Medical Association*, No. 7

Thapa, G P (1997), 'Women trafficking: better policing measures needed', *The Rising Nepal*, 15 July, Gorkhapatra Corporation Publication, Nepal

Tuladhar, J (1996), 'Social development in Nepal: gender perspective', in Maskey (ed), *Social Development in Nepal*, United Nations of Association of Nepal

UNICEF (1996), *Children and Women of Nepal: A Situation Analysis 1996*, UNICEF, Nepal

WHO/UNAIDS (1997), 'Epidemiological Fact Sheet on HIV/AIDS and Sexually Transmitted Diseases', WHO, Switzerland

Zierler, S and Krieger, N (1998), 'HIV infection in women: social inequalities as determinants of risk', *Critical Public Health*, Vol. 8, No.1

Gender, age, and exclusion:
a challenge to community organisations in Lima, Peru

Fiona C Clark and Nina Laurie

The designation of 1999 as the United Nations International Year for the Older Person has brought the issues of ageing and old age to the attention of policy-makers and governments. However, despite a series of recent international reports[1] which demonstrate growing awareness among international development organisations of the need to focus on elderly people worldwide, Peru's elderly population continues to be marginalised from formal support and is, therefore, increasingly dependent on informal social organisations to meet its needs.

'I am very sad to be here, I can't get used to it. Everything is very strange. I feel lost ... Now I don't eat properly, I don't have an appetite ... I don't know how to read or write, and because I am old and ill I can't work ... I live imprisoned in the house, I know nothing and no-one in the community ... If I do go out, I get lost, so my children won't let me out ... I am dependent on them.'
(Señora Mancario, elderly woman in her sixties from Tablada, Lima, Peru, 1996)

This article focuses on two successful grassroots women's organisations in Lima, Peru: the *Comedores Populares* (soup kitchens) and the *Vaso de Leche* (glass of milk) Programme. The *Comedores Populares* are predominantly locally organised and informal communal kitchens, which establish individual relationships with a variety of NGOs and charities (Vargas 1991). In contrast, the *Vaso de Leche* is a State-organised national programme, relying heavily on international food aid and political patronage. However, at the local level, both are run by women in their communities. The primary aim of both is poverty alleviation, specifically through improved nutrition. Through them, women have lobbied on issues such as provision of education and health services, and campaigned against the guerrilla insurgency of the 1980s and early 1990s (CENDOC MUJER 1991). However, we argue here that these organisations seem to have done little to include or empower women in old age. While the elderly were initially targeted by both, service provision for them has declined significantly over time. This is occurring at a point when economic adjustment and pension reform have made elderly people increasingly needy.

The article is based on information from three low-income settlements on the outskirts of Lima: Tablada de Lurin, San Juan de Dios, and Independencia. The work on which the article is based was carried out during two periods: the first, in 1996, lasted nine months and consisted of research into the inclusion of elderly people in social movements. Two years later, follow-up work consisted of examining the role of pension reform, and focused specifically on three clubs for elderly people. During these periods of data collection, we were assisted by having long-established relationships with a small, local Peruvian NGO which runs a range of community projects. Both the authors have long had an interest in women and social movements in Peru. Fiona Clark was a volunteer in this project in 1996, and Nina Laurie has collaborated with the organisation for eight years.

The ageing population in Peru

Endemic poverty still persists in Peru. It is particularly acute for older people, and especially indigenous women, who make up the largest proportion of the illiterate population in Peru. Of Peru's population of 25 million, just over one million (4.5 per cent) are aged over 65 (WDI 1998). Peru's elderly population has grown by 76 per cent since 1980, compared with an increase of 43 per cent for the population as a whole (ibid). This rise in the elderly population is occurring without an accompanying rise in affluence, thus creating an ever-larger, and poorer, sector of the population. The existing State social-security systems do not have the resources to satisfy the growing elderly population. Furthermore, the limited coverage of these formal systems leaves many still beyond the reach of social support programmes.

Elderly populations are 'feminised', in the sense that women's greater longevity means that they are a numerically dominant group among the very old (James 1998). In the elderly subset of the population[2] of Peru, men represent 45 per cent and women the other 55 per cent (WDI 1998), a sex ratio of 100 men to 122 women, compared with a sex ratio for the whole population of 100 men per 98 women. The age cohort over 80 shows an even greater imbalance. Elderly women are often more vulnerable than elderly men to economic instability in

old age, due to their comparatively limited access to education and employment earlier in life. They therefore face a number of barriers to securing assets for their old age.[3]

Gender and ageing in structural adjustment

In 1990, Peru became one of the few countries to introduce a programme of economic structural adjustment independent of the World Bank and the International Monetary Fund (IMF). Critics of economic structural adjustment policies have argued that these have a 'gender bias', and that because of this it is women who suffer more in times of austerity and economic rationalisation (Elson 1991). However, such analyses have seldom been extended to include women beyond child-bearing age. However, Peru's recent State and pension reforms and cutbacks in public-sector expenditures have affected spending on health and pension funds severely (Barrientos 1996), with particular consequences for women. In the past decade, reform to the pension system has aimed to make pensions economically sustainable. The main aim has been to remove the burden that they place on the State (James 1998, World Bank 1994), thus not extending their reach to poorer, less 'secure' investors.

While preliminary evidence suggests that this reform has been successful in achieving these particular aims (James 1998), it has failed to address prevailing biases against women, informal-sector workers, and rural dwellers that make it difficult for these groups to secure pensions. In 1994, 90.6 per cent of people aged 60 or over in Peru who received a State pension were men (INEI 1995).

'There are no services for the elderly here. The State doesn't provide social security for them. I worked in the haciendas (large farms) from the age of nine. Later I became a chauffeur

with a company, but they didn't pay enough, so I set up on my own ... then I had my car stolen, so I couldn't work any more. At the end of it all I had 43 credits[4] in my pension fund, and they (the social security) took away 30! They only pay me for 13, a pittance! They don't value my years of service. They've robbed me of my pension. I went to complain ... "A new system", they said. They were only counting the last 13 years! Then they took away my driving licence to make sure I didn't work again. The authorities really abuse people, there are many that should be receiving pensions and aren't getting a penny.' (Señor Perez, in his seventies, 1996)

Women, in particular, have difficulty in making pension contributions for the minimum period of 20 years, due to frequent gaps in formal employment, and low and unreliable income. A large proportion of women's paid and unpaid work is concentrated in informal-sector activities (Tanski 1994). In addition, it is typically interrupted by periods of child-birth and child-rearing. Furthermore, women are more likely than men to get non-monetary payment for their work (Grown and Sebstad 1987). All these factors make contributing to a pension very difficult.

As a result, many Peruvian women rely on their husbands' pensions, or on alternative methods of survival. Of those reliant on their spouses' pensions, 99.6 per cent were women (INEI 1995). On her husband's death, a widow receives a severely reduced survivor's pension of between 35 and 42 per cent of the pension for male employees. As Gorman (1995) suggests, 'for many women in developing countries the descent into total dependency begins with the death of the husband' (Gorman 1995, 121).

Exclusion within New Social Movements: two case studies

During the 1980s, the economic crisis suffered by much of Latin America provided the platform for the emergence of what came to be termed 'New Social Movements' (Escobar and Alvarez 1992). Increasingly desperate living conditions and severe poverty fuelled the growth of numerous small-scale, localised initiatives in the fight for daily survival. Lima has a long history of vibrant social movements, through which women and men have struggled to improve housing and address social needs in a context of urbanisation and increasing poverty (Moser and Peake 1987, Peattie 1990). These movements date back to the land invasions of the 1960s and 1970s, which created the *pueblos jovenes* (new towns) that emerged on the edge of the city (Lloyd 1980), and have since been the focus of much study. More recently, the *pueblos jovenes* have become famous as places where 'popular feminisms' have emerged, through the multitude of women's grassroots organisations that were established during the political and economic crises of the 1980s and early 1990s (Laurie et al 1997).

Peruvian women's activities at grassroots level have been seen as emblematic of the success of the New Social Movements, and have received much attention from researchers. The two organisations on which we focus here – the *Comedores Populares* and the *Vaso de Leche* Programme – were set up to meet basic needs. They have worked to alleviate poverty for two decades, and have been integral to community survival during this time. They are particularly noteworthy for their wide geographical and social coverage. The first *Comedores* began to appear in Lima at the start of the 1980s, when mothers started to pool food and money as part of household and community survival strategies. The *Vaso de Leche* scheme also started in this period, initially aiming to provide a ration of milk a day to children under six, pregnant women, and elderly people (El Sol 1996).

The following section examines how elderly people, and particularly women, are seen, and their interests and needs understood, by the *Comedores Populares* and the *Vaso de Leche*. It identifies the limited extent to which elderly women are included as beneficiaries and social actors.

The elderly: an unserved target group

'I used to receive milk from the Vaso de Leche. Now they don't include me any more. I don't get anything, not milk nor food at the Comedores. If my children don't give me any, I have nothing ... I am totally dependent on them.' (Señora Rosario, in her sixties, 1996)

Comedores seem to have excluded elderly community members in a number of contexts. Interviews with the *dirigentes* (leaders) of three elderly people's clubs in Tablada, Independencia, and San Juan de Dios revealed that none of them had successfully managed to obtain support from the local *Comedores* for their members, despite having asked for it repeatedly. In 1996, Tablada had 62 *Comedores Populares* (Gamarra 1996), and, while 81 per cent of the 35 elderly people interviewed from this area mentioned having the facility of a soup kitchen near them, only 23 per cent of this group said they used it regularly. Nineteen per cent said they used it occasionally, while the rest did not use it at all. In Independencia, none of the 28 members of the old people's club had access to a *Comedor*, and in San Juan de Dios, only two out of 40 members were given rations as 'special cases'.[5] The club in San Juan de Dios did manage to arrange for

the local municipality to allow six group members to eat free in the municipal *Comedores*. However, this *Comedor* was located in central Independencia – a 10-minute bus-ride or half-hour walk away – and the six members were not able to take up the offer, because they could not manage the long walk up and down a steep hill, nor afford the daily return bus fare.

The national *Vaso de Leche* programme initially included the elderly among its target groups. However, recent cuts in milk rations, related to the funding crisis caused by the retraction of most foreign aid during the civil war, and subsequent government cuts in welfare expenditure, had the inevitable outcome that the little milk that remained was channelled to children and pregnant mothers. The ration for the elderly was the first to be reduced. As a consequence, in Tablada, 31 per cent of older people interviewed reported having been withdrawn from the programme. Some centres are even explicit in their exclusion of elderly people from the programme:

'Even the Vaso de Leche hasn't given me any help. I went and said to them: "Please, I too need milk", but they said: "No, not for old women. This is for babies, for the little ones."... They clearly told me that the Vaso de Leche was only for children. I even stood in the doorway waiting for left-overs, and they still didn't give me any.' (Señora Huamán, in her sixties, 1998)

Even those who previously received help from centres when these first started reported that they now received very little:

'When I arrived from the mountains (1991) they gave me a whole bag full of milk – a whole bag. Now they give so little.' (Señora Vega, in her fifties, 1996)

Explaining the exclusion of elderly people

One of the reasons for neglect of elderly women and men is that both the *Comedores Populares* and the *Vaso de Leche* programme, like most poverty-alleviation programmes, register households rather than individuals. Eligibility of a household for inclusion on either of the programmes is based on the number of children per household, in an attempt to combat child malnutrition. This automatically excludes any households without children and potentially neglects and renders invisible elderly people living in poverty.

Poverty analyses that focus on the household do the elderly no favours, since they 'misrepresent intra-household behaviour, obscure intra-household stratification by gender and generation, and stifle the voices of the unempowered' (Wolfe 1990, 44). They also hide the contributions of older people to the care and maintenance of the household, and therefore overlook their right as active household members to benefit from the activities of social movements that aim to support this work. Where grandparents are present in the family, they tend to be perceived as non-active household members who live in 'a situation of complete passivity' (INEI 1995, 13) as victims of their age. Even when elderly women (and men) do contribute actively to the income of the household, this type of work is often invisible and not valued, even by the elderly themselves. Elia Luna, in charge of establishing one programme in Lima attending to elderly people, states:

'Frequently an elderly woman, when asked if she "works" will reply "no", even though she spends most of her day selling vegetables or fruit in the market, or selling home-prepared food in the street. ... This is a problem in society – that this kind of informal work is not given the value it deserves and is not seen as "work".' (Elia Luna, Lima, 1998)

Conventional perceptions of the elderly as passive dependants makes their exclusion from the benefits of the *Comedores Populares* and *Vaso de Leche* more likely, since both organisations use a rhetoric of temporary assistance and self-help, rather than welfare. *Comedores* have a clear remit to provide temporary support to families for one or two months, to help them to 'get back on their feet' until they find work, or other means to support themselves. Although the *Vaso de Leche* initially intended to target the elderly as well as children, it actually aims in the main to reduce infant malnutrition, and help the growth of children in their first years of life. While the temporary nature of such support remains mainly rhetorical (during the 1980s and early 1990s these organisations provided long-term welfare – see Laurie 1995), extending assistance to the elderly is resisted, because there can be little doubt that for many this support is likely to be needed until they die.

Not only have the organisations excluded the elderly as a vulnerable group, but they have also failed to recognise the crucial support that many elderly women give them, both directly and indirectly. Literature and popular opinion has celebrated the role of young women as mothers in the success of *Comedores Populares* and the *Vaso de Leche* (see, for example, CENDOC MUJER 1991), but these women do not necessarily have the time to participate fully in the running of the organisations. Elderly women may take over the household tasks while their daughters contribute time to the *Comedores Populares* or *Vaso de Leche* programmes, or participate themselves. One young single mother described how her mother fetches and distributes milk for the *Vaso de Leche* programme:

'In comité *number six, there is nothing but arguments: "I don't have time to go, you should go" ... The only one who goes (to pick up the milk) is my mother...[with] the neighbour,*

while the other women are there sitting idle with their husbands and children, and don't help with even one glass of milk. All her life my mother has gone and fetched the milk, ever since the centre opened, while other (younger) Señoras sit and complain that "no, I can't go because I have to look after my children, I can't go because I've too much to do"' ... And my mother? I suppose she doesn't have anything better to do? She, as it happens, has to look after her grandchildren, because her daughters are out working.' (Señora Gomez, younger single mother, Tablada, Lima, Peru 1996)

Señora Gomez's words challenge an important assumption about the *Vaso de Leche* and other women's organisations like it. This is that they 'empower' women and relieve them of their drudgery: in fact, they may place an extra burden on the very women whom they are meant to target and who already face a heavy workload. Under such circumstances, the running and continued 'success' of these programmes very often relies on the work of the very household members (the elderly) who are excluded from their direct benefits.

To summarise, no long-term support is available from these organisations to promote the welfare of elderly people. Second, the contribution that elderly members of households make to the work of the organisations is invisible and undervalued. Therefore, even in the most successful New Social Movements in Lima, rather than being seen as social actors and citizens in their own right, elderly people are often perceived as non-priority and passive members of society in need of 'charity'.

'Self-help': an alternative to social movements?

A number of *Clubes de Tercer Edad* (elderly people's clubs), focusing exclusively on the needs of the elderly,

have emerged in Lima in recent years. The impetus to set them up often comes from the recognition that elderly people have no alternative to self-help, due to their exclusion from long-standing social movements: in many cases, the very social movements that, as younger people, they helped to organise. While feminist literature has heralded the success of organisations such as the *Comedores Populares* and the *Vaso de Leche* in providing strategic opportunities for low-income women (Barrig 1989, Galter and Nuñez 1989), the role-loss and isolation experienced by elderly women who were once their founders have not been acknowledged.

'I have always been in the Vaso de Leche *and the* Comedores, *but once I got older and started not feeling so well, I had to withdraw from my activities. I felt very poorly and so I had to stop. So now I am sat here, stuck in my house, I am very lonely. I had got used to always mixing with local people and having contact with local institutions. Now I've been left feeling very alone, uncomfortable. It really hit me hard, and I was very depressed. I saw myself getting worse because I wasn't participating any more. So that's when I decided to form my own group of Señoras like me, a group for elderly people. So since 1993, my husband and I have been working on this – working – but still we receive no help, and yet every day I see more elderly people [who are] ... lonely.* (Señora Castro, a woman in her seventies, Independencia, Lima, Peru 1998)

The groups have met with varied success in terms of providing for the nutritional needs of their members. For example, while one club failed to establish workable links with a local *Comedor*, it has been more successful with the *Vaso de Leche*, which now gives the group 12 bags of milk and seven bags of oats each week. It is important, however, not to over-estimate the extent of this help, as each individual receives a ration of two bags of milk and one of oats – a weekly ration for the usual recipient of the *Vaso de Leche* – only every six to seven weeks.

A gender analysis of exclusion

Mainstream development policy has concentrated too much on 'developing' people in the productive part of their life cycle, and this has tended to marginalise elderly people from development programmes and agendas. More specifically, feminist analyses of development have tended to focus almost entirely on young, often single, metropolitan women and their involvement in employment and social movements, at the expense of including older, 'provincial' women (Laurie 1999). Such analyses have failed to acknowledge the cumulative effect of social, economic, and political biases against women throughout their life course, or the impact this has on their well-being in old age.

The desire of the elderly to do something to meet their own needs could be seen in the same positive light as feminists and gender and development workers saw the early self-help housing movements of the 1970s, or the opportunities afforded to young women leaders who started the soup kitchens in the 1980s. On the other hand, we could also see it as proof of the failure of the New Social Movements to adapt to the changing needs of the communities in which they work. These movements, set up to meet basic needs, seem to have been unable to incorporate difference between members, or to create fluid institutional structures and targets capable of meeting the needs of ageing members.

Despite the fact that elderly women are 'likely to suffer problems accruing not only from present abandonment, but also from earlier disadvantage' (Tout 1989, 289),

elderly women seem to be an invisible group in feminist debates in Peru. For example, a leading Limeñan feminist organisation said *'we deal with women, not with elderly people'*, when they were contacted concerning the research for this project. Why is it that contemporary debates on gender and development in Peru have not addressed the issue of elderly women? One of the reasons suggested by an activist on issues of old age in Tablada is the fact that few older women themselves have reflected upon their gendered experience of poverty:

'The majority of women have not thought about their gender roles or how this affects their life. They will tell you how much they suffered and how hard they have had to work, but they will say "I suffered because I am poor", rather than "I suffered because I am poor and a woman".' (Mili Castro, leader of club for elderly people, 1998)

It would appear that, despite more than three decades of active middle-class and 'popular' feminisms, there is a generation of women, now of advancing years, who have not yet had the opportunity to reflect on their experience of poverty and discrimination, or to understand it as anything more than class-based.

Conclusion

This article has pointed out that the ageing of Latin American populations is an issue that has to be taken seriously very soon. Social security systems are currently faced with the challenge of a growing elderly population, which is predominantly female. In Peru, the privatisation of the pension system has highlighted the inherent gender, urban, and formal-economy biases that continue to exclude many people, and especially women, from its benefits. The Peruvian State should not rely on the family, or social movements, to compensate for inadequate government social security provision. The State, in partnership with international agencies, NGOs, and community leaders, must recognise and value the existing and potential work of elderly members of the community, to enable the elderly to play a part in their own welfare provision.

Researchers and policy-makers need to look more closely at the position of elderly women and men within the poverty debates, and gender and development debates, if the complexities of exclusion in later life are to be understood. This shift in policy focus is necessary if older people, and especially women, are to be given a voice that allows them to discuss the ageing process and bring ageism into the open, so that it can be countered. A gender analysis of opportunities through the life course makes for a better understanding of the particular obstacles facing women in old age. Today's old people represent the future of almost everyone, and every country. As such, ageing has to be acknowledged as a real development challenge, rather than the elderly person being perceived as the 'antithesis' of development (Gorman 1995).

Fiona Clark is a consultant for the Latin American and Caribbean Region's Social Development Department of the World Bank, Washington, DC. 1818 H Street, Washington, DC 20433, USA. E-mail: fclark@worldbank.org

Nina Laurie is a Lecturer in Human Geography at the University of Newcastle upon Tyne, UK. Department of Geography, University of Newcastle upon Tyne, Claremont Road, Newcastle upon Tyne, NE1 7RU, UK. E-mail: nina.laurie@newcastle.ac.uk

Notes

1 Reports have come from the UK Department for International Development (DfID 1999), HelpAge International (HAI 1995), INSTRAW (1999), the United Nations Population Fund (UNFPA 1998), and the World Bank (1994).

2 Those over the age of 65.

3 For a wider discussion of gender-based economic exclusion, see Clark (1999). For a discussion of women over the life course, see Pratt and Hanson (1995).

4 One credit is equal to one year's service.

5 One elderly woman receives a daily meal for her and her husband because her husband is paralysed. The other elderly woman receives food for herself and her children because she works (unremunerated) in the *Comedores* every day from eight a.m. until three p.m.

References

Barrientos, A (1996), 'Pension reform and pension coverage in Chile: lessons for other countries', in *Bulletin of Latin American Research*, Vol.15, No.3

Barrig, M (1989), 'The difficult equilibrium between bread and roses: women's organisations and the transition from dictatorship to democracy in Peru', in Jaquette (ed.), *The Women's Movement in Latin America and the Transition to Democracy*, Unwin Hyman, USA

CENDOC MUJER (1991), *El Movimiento popular de Mujeres como Respuesta a la Crisis*, CENDOC MUJER, Peru

Clark, F C (1999), 'Old age, gender and marginality in Peru: development for the elderly', in *Ageing in a Gendered World: Women's Issues and Identities*, INSTRAW, Dominican Republic, INSTRAW/Ser.B/53

DFID (1999), *Ageing and Development* by Alison Heslop, Working paper No. 3, Social Development Department, Department for International Development, UK

El Sol (1996), *Se vienen cambios en Vaso de Leche*, Lima, 13 May 1996

88

Elson, D (ed.) (1991), *Male Bias in the Development Process*, Manchester University Press, UK

Escobar, A and Alvarez, S E (1992), *The Making of Latin American Social Movements: Identity, Strategy and Democracy*, Westview Press, USA

Galter, N and Nuñez, P (1989), *Mujer y Comedores Populares*, SEPADE, Peru

Gamarra Garcia, H (1996), 'Informe de Servicio Rural Urbano Marginal de Salud', unpublished, Peru

Gorman, M (1995), 'Older people and development : the last minority?', in *Development in Practice*, Vol. 5, No.2, Oxfam, UK

Grown, C and Sebstad, J (1989), 'Introduction: towards a wider perspective of women's employment', *World Development*, Vol. 17, No. 7

Help Age International (1995), *Older Women in Development* (ed. Katrina Payne), Help Age International, UK

INEI (1995), *Peru, Perfil socio-demográfico de la Tercer Edad*, Peru

INSTRAW (1999), *Ageing in a Gendered World: Women's Issues and Identities*, INSTRAW, Dominican Republic, INSTRAW/Ser.B/53

James, E (1998), 'Pension reform in Latin America: is there an efficiency-equity trade-off?' in Bridsall, Graham, and Sabot (eds), *Beyond Trade-offs: Market Reforms and Equitable Growth in Latin America*, IDB and Brookings Press:USA

Laurie, N (1995), 'Negotiating Gender: Women and Emergency Employment in Peru', unpublished PhD thesis, University of London, UK

Laurie, N (1997), 'Negotiating femininity: women and representation in emergency employment in Peru', in *Gender, Place and Culture*, Vol. 4, No. 2

Laurie, N (1999), 'Negotiating femininities in the "provinces": women and emergency employment in Peru', *Environment and Planning 'A'* , Vol. 31, No. 2

Laurie, N et al (1997), 'In and out of bounds and resisting boundaries: feminist geographies of space and place', in WGSG, *Feminist Geographies: Explorations in Diversity and Difference*, Longman, London

Lloyd, P (1980), *The Young Towns of Lima: Aspects of Urbanisation in Peru*, Cambridge University Press, UK

Moser, C and Peake, L (1987), *Women, Human Settlements and Housing*, Tavistock Publications, UK

Peattie, L (1990), 'Participation: a case study of how invaders organise, negotiate and interact with government in Lima, Peru', in *Environment and Urbanisation*, Vol. 2, No.19

Pratt, G and Hanson, S (1995), 'Gender, work and space', in Katz and Monk, *Full Circles: Geographies of Women over the Life Course*, Routledge, UK

Tanski, J M (1994), 'The impact of crisis, stabilisation and structural adjustment on women in Lima, Peru', *World Development*, Vol. 22, No.11

Tout, K (1989), *Ageing in Developing Countries*, Help Age International, Oxford University Press, UK

UNFPA (1998), *The State of the World's Population 1998. The New Generations*, UNFPA, USA

Vargas, V (1991), 'The women's movement in Peru: streams, spaces and knots', *European Review of Latin American and Caribbean Studies*, No. 50

WDI (World Development Indicators) (1998), *World Development Database*, World Bank, USA

Wolfe, D (1990), 'Daughters' decisions and domination: an empirical and conceptual critique of household strategies', *Development and Change*, No. 21

World Bank (1994), *Averting the Old Age Crisis: Policies to protect the old and promote growth*, Oxford University Press, UK

Resources

Compiled by Erin Murphy Graham

Gender and ageing

The Ageing and Development Report: Poverty, Independence, and the World's Older People (1999), HelpAge International, Earthscan Publications, 120 Pentonville Road, London N1 9JN, UK.

The first extensive survey of older people in the developing world, including economic issues, health systems, work, and family relationships. The first section presents an introduction to ageing and development. The second presents regional information on the State of the World's Older People. The third part presents data on Ageing and Development, and the fourth has references, with lists of member organisations of HelpAge International.

Women, Ageing and Health: Achieving Health across the Life Span (1996), R. Bonita, World Health Organisation, Distribution and Sales, CH- 1211, Geneva 27, Switzerland. E-mail: publications@who.ch; fax (41) 22 791 4857.

Global in its approach, the report identifies certain health needs shared by all ageing women, discusses their determinants, and then shows how these needs can be met through cost-effective strategies.

Older Women in Development (1995), HelpAge International, 3rd Floor, 67–74 Saffron Hill, London EC1N 8QX, UK.

This booklet includes brief case studies from Ghana, Peru, India, Chile, Tanzania, Grenada, Costa Rica, and Rwanda. It relates issues of ageing to poverty, work, caring and health services, emergencies, and education.

A World of Widows (1996), Margaret Owen, Zed Books, 7 Cynthia Street, London N1 9FJ, UK.

Widowhood, on an international level, is explored in this volume. Issues addressed include the process of becoming a widow, differing laws regarding inheritance, widows who remarry, and sexuality and health. The book concludes with a summary of widowhood as a human-rights issue, and an overview of what widows are doing to organise for change.

Gender Issues in Elder Abuse (1996), Lynda Aitken and Gabriele Griffen, Sage Publications, 6 Bonhill Street, London EC2A 4PU.

This book analyses the ways in which gender is central to the occurrence, detection, and prevention of abuse of the elderly.

AGEWAYS: Practical Agecare for Development, HelpAge International, 67–74 Saffron Hill, London EC1N 8QX, UK. AGEWAYS is a quarterly journal dedicated to the issues of ageing and age-care in developing countries. Also published in Spanish as *HORIZONTES: Ayuda a la Ancianidad para el Desarrollo.*

Ageing and Development, HelpAge International. This journal, published three times a year, aims to raise awareness of the contribution, needs, and rights of older people, and to promote the development of laws and policies supporting older people.

The girl-child

The State of the World's Children 2000 (2000), UNICEF, United Nations Publications, E-mail: info@unicef.org.uk fax (44) 020 7405 2332
Since 1979, this annual series has drawn international attention to the challenges facing children and has pressed for sustained action to protect and promote their well-being. The most recent report issues an urgent call to leadership on behalf of children and discusses four of the most daunting obstacles to development: poverty, violence, disease, and discrimination.

Traditional and Cultural Practices Harmful to the Girl-Child (1997), African Centre for Women Occasional Paper No. 1, Economic Commission for Africa (ECA), Development Information Services Division, UNECAP, PO Box 3001, Addis Ababa, Ethiopia.
This booklet discusses practices that are harmful to girls yet are perpetuated or ignored, due to ignorance or cultural tradition. Examples are drawn from countries in Africa to illustrate these problems. The last section contains policy recommendations.

Programming for Adolescent Health and Development: Report of a WHO/UNFPA/ UNICEF Study Group on Programming for Adolescent Health (1999), World Health Organisation, Technical Report Series, No. 886.
The report aims to establish a framework of strategies and principles that can support programmes for adolescent health at country level, particularly in the developing world. The report draws on practical experiences and recent research findings to reach conclusions on which interventions work best.

Adolescent Health: Reassessing the Passage to Adulthood (1995), Judith Senderowitz, World Bank Discussion Papers No. 272. 1818 H Street, NW, Washington, DC 20043, USA.
This paper discusses the slow development of programmes to meet adolescents' health needs in developing countries, and reviews the current data on adolescent health, with an emphasis on reproductive and sexual activity. It argues that gender discrimination in food allocation, health-care and education compromises young women's current and future well-being. It also highlights the greater health risks faced by adolescent females because of factors related to reproduction, including early pregnancy and childbearing.

Trafficking and exploitation of children

The Prostitution of Women and Girls (1998), R Barri Flowers, McFarland & Company Inc. Publishers, Box 611, Jefferson, North Carolina 28640, USA.
This book explores the complex issues surrounding the prostitution of women and girls internationally. The third part examinesthe extent of teenage prostitution, the characteristics of girl prostitutes, runaway girls, and the dimensions and dangers of child sexual abuse.

Kids for Hire: A Child's Right to Protection from Commercial Sexual Exploitation (1996), Save the Children, Mary Datchelor House, 17 Grove Lane, London SE5 8RD, UK.

Kids for Hire looks into various ways in which the problem of sexually exploited children can be addressed by development organisations, focusing its attention on six areas: good information and research, prevention, protection, rehabilitation, co-ordination among NGOs, and the participation of the children themselves in addressing the issue. Brief case studies are included on children from Vietnam, Cambodia, Philippines, Brazil, Honduras, and the UK.

The Human Rights Watch Global Report on Women's Human Rights (1995), Human Rights Watch, 33 Islington High Street, N1 9LH, London, UK.

A compilation of investigations by Human Right Watch from 1990 to 1995 is presented in this volume. Several case studies are included on the forced prostitution, coerced marriage, and trafficking of women and girls in South and South-East Asia. General recommendations to governments, the United Nations, and donor countries are included.

Wish You Weren't Here: The Sexual Exploitation of Children and the Connection with Tourism and International Travel (1993), Kevin Ireland, Save the Children, Mary Datchelor House, 17 Grove Lane, London SE5 8RD, UK.

This report attempts to explore the links between international tourism and the sexual abuse and exploitation of children by tourists and international travellers. The last section of the report presents intervention strategies, including international co-operation, and argues that action must be taken within countries of tourist origin.

Disposable People: New Slavery in the Global Economy (1999), Kevin Bales, University of California Press, 1600 Hershey Hall, 610 Young Drive, University of California, Los Angeles, CA 90095-1373, USA.

Drawing on case studies from Thailand, Mauritania, Brazil, Pakistan, and India, this volume explores modern-day slavery and what can be done to end it. The last section focuses on what can be done to stop slavery, and offers five specific actions that individuals can take.

Street Children: Struggling Against the Odds (1992), World Association of Girl Guides and Girl Scouts, 12c Lyndhurst Road, London NW3 5PQ, UK.

This booklet contains a brief introduction to the problems of street children, stressing that street children are not just found in developing countries, but in European cities. Street girls are among the most vulnerable and exploited of all street children. Profiles of street girls from Manila, Brazil, and London are included, as well as information about projects to help street girls in the UK, Philippines, USA, Brazil, Peru, and Rwanda.

Street and Working Children: A Guide to Planning (1994), Save the Children.

This manual is relevant for both researchers and those working directly with street children. It argues that over the past decade street children have received increased attention because of tourism, international press coverage, and films or documentaries, and that many inter-national development agencies have based successful fundraising campaigns on images of street children. Compared with street children, working children do not receive the same response, despite the fact that millions of them work in agriculture, workshops, and factories, and as domestic servants. The manual includes chapters on carrying out first-hand research, project options, common problems, and suggested solutions.

Child Labour – An Information Kit for Teachers, Educators and their Organisations (1998), International Labour Organisation, 1211 GENEVA 22 Switzerland. Fax: +41 22 799 8578; email: publns@ilo.org; Internet: http://www.ilo.org/publns

The kit aims to assist teachers, educators, and their organisations in carrying out actions and campaigns against child labour. The kit contains information, and examples of practical tools for use in the classroom and the community. The first book, gives facts and figures on child labour and underlines the importance of education in the elimination of child labour. The second book is a collection of successful initiatives from 13 countries, showing how various groups around the world have worked to solve child-labour problems through educational programmes.

Child Soldiers: The Role of Children in Armed Conflict (1997), Ilene Cohn and Guy S Goodwin-Gill, Oxford University Press, Great Clarendon Street, Oxford OX2 6DP, UK.

This book assesses the status of children soldiers in international law. It discusses why children participate in armed conflict, and the conditions and consequences of their participation. It concludes with a series of recommendations to prevent recruitment and calls for the creation of a more coherent policy of treatment for children who have participated in violent conflict.

Children: the Invisible Soldiers (1996), Radda Barnen, Swedish Save the Children, 107 88 Stockholm, Sweden.

Based on case studies from 26 countries, this report, commissioned by the UN Study on the Impact of Armed Conflict on Children, documents how and why children become soldiers. Special attention is given to gender issues.

HIV/AIDS, age, and gender

The Hidden Cost of AIDS: The Challenge of HIV to Development (1992), The Panos Institute, 9 White Lion Street, London N1 9PD, UK.

This book provides a general overview of the economic, demographic, and social implications of HIV/AIDS throughout the developing world, with a special focus on sub-Saharan Africa. Chapter Four focuses on the social costs of HIV/AIDS in the community. This chapter also examines the ways in which women are disproportionately affected by the HIV/AIDS epidemic.

The Looming Epidemic: The Impact of HIV and AIDS in India (1998), Peter Goodwin (ed) Hurst & Company, 38 King Street, London WC2E 8JZ, UK.

A collection of reports of research findings, analytical frameworks, and suggestions for future research are included in this volume on HIV/AIDS in India. The last chapter focuses on 'Gender Differentials and the Special Vulnerability of Women', which, while discussed within the Indian context, is also relevant in other settings. Additional attention is given to the importance of the needs of children and AIDS orphans.

Children Orphaned by AIDS: Frontline Responses from Eastern and Southern Africa (1999), UNICEF Publications, 55 Lincoln's Inn Fields, WC2A 3NB London, UK.

This report discusses the impact of AIDS, beyond the deaths of millions of people, focusing on the children who lose one or both parents to the AIDS virus. It argues that by the end of 2000 a cumulative total of 1.3 million children will have lost their parents. It examines how the AIDS epidemic affects children, and offers policy recommendations for individual countries to help affected children.

Researching life stories

Researching Life Stories and Family Histories (2000), Robert L. Miller, Sage Publications, 6 Bonhill Street, London EC2A 4PU, UK.
This book covers the main methods and issues in collecting and analysing life histories. It also includes exercises to help master these methodologies.

Listening for A Change: Oral Testimony and Development (1993), Hugo Slim and Paul Thompson, Panos Publications.
This book was published as part of the Panos Oral Testimony Programme. People want to speak for themselves, and not to be heard through the distorting medium of outside 'experts'. Using case studies from around the world, it illustrates the different ways in which aid agencies – and communities themselves – can use oral history.

Oral History: A Handbook (1998), Ken Wowarth. Sutton Publishing, Phoenix Mill, Gloucestershire G15 2BU, UK.
This book offers a broad discussion of oral history, from the philosophical to the practical. It includes chapters on interview planning and recording, storage of media, and the use of video. It ends with a section on 'using oral history', and also includes appendices with sample questions and guidance on ethical issues.

At the Desert's Edge: Oral Histories from the Sahel (1991). Nigel Cross and Rhiannon Barker (eds.), Panos Publications.
This collection of oral histories is an example of the power of this method of finding out about people. It offers the life-stories of more than 500 men and women in eight Sahelian countries.

Three Generations, Two Genders, One World (1998), Sylvia Chant and Cathy McIlwaine (editors), Zed Books.
This fascinating book is the outcome of a multi-country oral history research project undertaken by students with their own family members. The project was instigated by the Commonwealth Secretariat prior to the UN Women's Conference in Beijing, 1995. It looked at shifts in the values, attitudes, relationships and gender roles of three generations of women and men, in nine countries in South and North. The contextual differences are highlighted, together with the striking similarities in what it means to be male and female in our 'globalising' world.

Organisations

UNICEF, UNICEF House, 3 United Nations Plaza, New York, New York 10017, USA.
Http://www.unicef.org/
Email addresses@unicef.org
Founded in 1946, UNICEF advocates and works for the protection of children's rights, to help the young to meet their basic needs and to expand their opportunities to reach their full potential. UNICEF is guided by the Convention on the Rights of the Child and strives to establish children's rights as enduring ethical principles and international standards of behaviour towards children.

Save the Children (International Save the Children Alliance), 275-281 King Street, London W6 9LZ, UK.
Tel: +44 20 8748 2554; fax: +44 20 8237 8000
Http://www.savethechildren.net/newstc/
Email: info@save-children-alliance.org
Since 1919, Save the Children has been working to promote the rights and improve living conditions of children around the world. Working in more than 100 countries across the globe and comprising 26 organisations, Save the Children also works with mothers, recognising that 'when mothers thrive, children thrive', and has recently published a report on The State of the World's Mothers.

PLAN International, 5-6 Underhill Street, London NW1 7HS, UK.
Tel: 020 7485 6612; fax: 020 7485 2107
Http://www.plan-international.org/uk/home.html
PLAN International is a child-focused development organisation that, for more than 60 years, has helped millions of children, and their families, throughout the world. PLAN International now works in 14 donor countries (including the UK) and in over 40 programme countries, with more than one million sponsored children world-wide

Street Kids International, 398 Adelaide St. W, Suite 1000, 10th floor, Toronto, Canada M5V 1S7.
Tel: 416 504 8994; fax: 416 504 8977.
Http://www.streetkids.org/about.html
E-mail ski@streetkids.org
Street Kids International works to help those who work with street kids at the local level: front-line workers who can respect their individuality, understand their dilemmas, and create opportunities for them to build better lives. Street Kids International attempts to help street children by creating and sharing innovative approaches to both urgent needs and underlying causes.

International Programme on the Elimination of Child Labour (IPEC), International Labour Organisation.
Tel: +41.22.799.8181; fax: +41.22.799.8771.
Http://www.ilo.org/public/english/standards/ipec/index.htm,
E-Mail: ipec@ilo.org
The aim of IPEC is to work towards the progressive elimination of child labour by strengthening national capacities to address child-labour problems, and by creating a world-wide movement to combat it. The priority target groups are bonded child labourers, children in hazardous working conditions and occupations, very young working children and working girls.

HelpAge International (Help the Aged), 67–74 Saffron Hill, London EC1N 8QX, UK.
Tel: +44 171 404 7201; fax: +44 171 404 7203
http://www.helpage.org/index.html;
e-mail: hai@helpage.org
HelpAge International is a development agency that works through a network of development, research, and community-based and social-service organisations that share the goal of improving the lives of disadvantaged older people. Founded in 1983 as an independent charity by HelpAge India, Help the Aged Canada, Pro Vida Colombia, HelpAge Kenya, and Help the Aged UK, it has grown to include the present membership of 62 organisations world-wide.

The International Institute on Ageing, United Nations-Malta, 117 St Paul Street, Valletta VLT 07 Malta.
Tel: 2430044/5/6; fax: 230248
http://www.inia.org.mt/;
email: inia@maltanet.net
The main objectives of the Institute on Ageing are to fulfil the training needs of developing countries and to facilitate the implementation of the Vienna International Plan of Action on Ageing. The Institute provides multi-disciplinary education and training in specific areas related to ageing, and also acts as a catalyst as regards the exchange of information on issues concerned with ageing.

UNAIDS, 20 Avenue Appia, CH-1211 Geneva 27, Switzerland.
Tel: (+4122) 791 3666; fax: (+4122) 791 4187
http://www.unaids.org
email: unaids@unaids.org
The mission of UNAIDS is to lead, strengthen, and support an expanded response to the AIDS epidemic that will prevent the spread of HIV, provide care and support for those infected and affected by the disease, reduce the vulnerability of individuals and communities to HIV/AIDS, and alleviate the socio-economic and human impact of the epidemic.

Websites

World Health Organisation Ageing and Health Programme
http://www.who.int/ageing/index.html
In April 1995, WHO launched a new programme on Ageing and Health. This website highlights the programmes in several focus areas, including life course, health promotion, culture, and gender. The purpose of the programme is to promote health and well-being throughout the life span, thus ensuring the highest possible level of quality of life for as long as possible, for the largest possible number of older people.

Global Movement for Active Ageing
http://www.who.int/ageing/global_movement/index.html
The Global Movement for Active Ageing, which was conceived by the World Health Organisation, acts as a network for all those who are interested in moving policies and practice towards 'Active Ageing', or the capacity of people, as they grow older, to lead productive and healthy lives in their families, societies and economies. The key messages of the movement are the celebration of ageing, the recognition that older persons can continue to contribute to a society for all, and the promotion of intergenerational solidarity. This site also contains models and ideas for programmes and projects that promote active ageing.

Pan-American Health Organisation Unit on Ageing and Health
http://www.paho.org/english/hpp/hee-index.htm
The unit on Ageing and Health in the Family Health and Population Programme of the Division of Health Promotion and Protection aims to promote public and health policies with a focus on active ageing, promote the health and well-being of older persons, and encourage initiatives to create health promotion and disease-prevention interventions for older persons.

International Labour Organisation: Child Labour
http://www.ilo.org/public/english/comp/child/
This website contains information on the ILO policy on child labour, international law, and links to publications on child labour. Its 'news room' contains information kits, video and audio clips, posters and photographs, and relevant articles from the ILO publication, World of Work.

UNICEF
http://www.unicef.org/
UNICEF's homepage has useful links to publications, the Convention on the Rights of the Child, and UNICEF programmes and activities. Voices of Youth, a discussion-based site hosted by UNICEF where young people are encouraged to express their opinions on current issues, is one of these programmes (http://www.unicef.org/voy/). In addition, there is a list of links to other organisations that work to prevent child labour, and papers on child labour:
Oneworld's Big Issues: Child Labour
http://www.oneworld.org/guides/chld_labour/index.html

Child Rights Information Network (CRIN)
http://www.crin.org
CRIN is a global network of organisations exchanging information about children's rights to promote the UN Convention on the Rights of the Child and to improve policy and practice of organisations around the world. This website is a valuable resource on the implementation and monitoring of the Convention. It also includes bibliographic references, databases, a calendar of events, and links to other child-focused sites.

The Girl Child Working Group: WomenWatch Beijing + 5 Global Forum
http://www.un.org/womenwatch/for/girl/girl.htm#top

This site has detailed information on the Platform for Action adopted at the Beijing Conference in 1995, which defined nine strategic objectives for the girl-child. The Girl Child Working Group homepage discusses how these strategic objectives have been met and what lessons have been learned in efforts to achieve these goals.

Children and Aids International Non-Government Organisation Network (CAINN)
http://www.pedhivaids.org/education/children_living.html
The CAINN network was established in 1996 by NGOs and community-based organisations to promote the voices, rights, and needs of children and young people infected by, affected by, and vulnerable to HIV/AIDS. Its key objective is to promote the implementation of the UN Convention on Rights of the Child and other relevant international declarations and agreements.

Videos

Karate Kids (1989), Street Kids International
See contact information above
This animated video story serves as a discussion tool, aimed at 8–14 year olds, about HIV/AIDS prevention and sexual health issues. It attempts to encourage young people to ask questions about street life and sexually transmitted diseases. It is available in 23 languages and is currently used by youth workers in more than 100 countries.

The following videos are available from UNICEF (see contact information above). More information is available at http://www.unicef.org

The State of the World's Children, 1997 (1996)
This 1997 video report consists of succinct video news items that accompany the report published every year. The video report includes short stories for timely news leads, statements by UNICEF's Executive Director, and B-roll footage. The State of the World's Children 1997 video calls for an immediate end to hazardous and exploitative child labour. Featured are testimonials from working children – bonded child labourers in India's bidi (cigarette) industry, street beggars in Senegal and under-age garment workers in Bangladesh – that illustrate the appalling conditions endured by millions of children each day.

Rights of Passage (1994)
This film depicts the hardship and challenges faced by four girls reaching adolescence in Burkina Faso, India, Jamaica, and Nicaragua. It presents a sensitive and personal portrayal of their lives and the issues of drug abuse, teenage pregnancy, education discrimination, and female genital mutilation – problems faced by many girls around the world.

Soldier Boy (1997), UNICEF and Danish TV
This film depicts the tragic consequences of violence for the lives of children in Liberia, West Africa, where thousands of children aged seven or over are fighting as soldiers in a civil war that began in 1989. One quarter of the combatants are children.

Dream Girls (1996)
This documentary follows four girls living on the streets of Rio de Janeiro, Brazil, three of whom make their living through prostitution.

In Uganda, Caring for Children Orphaned by Aids
Video clip in Real format available at http://www.unicef.org/pon99/video.htm
In Uganda today, a stunning 11 per cent of the total child population are now AIDS orphans. Grandparents are playing a leading role in supporting children orphaned by AIDS.